Second Edition

THERAPEUTIC EXERCISE

FOR BODY ALIGNMENT AND FUNCTION

LUCILLE DANIELS, M.A.
Professor of Physical Therapy, Emerita,
School of Medicine, Stanford University

CATHERINE WORTHINGHAM, Ph.D., D.Sc.
Formerly, Director of Professional Education,
The National Foundation, Inc.

Illustrations by
Harold Black, Lorene Sigal and Phyllis Hedberg

W. B. SAUNDERS COMPANY
PHILADELPHIA • LONDON • TORONTO • 1977

W. B. Saunders Company: West Washington Square
Philadelphia, Pa.   19105

1 St. Anne's Road
Eastbourne, East Sussex BN21 3UN, England

1 Goldthorne Avenue
Toronto, Ontario M8Z 5T9, Canada

Library of Congress Cataloging in Publication Data

Daniels, Lucille.
  Therapeutic exercise for body alignment and function.

1. Exercise therapy.   2. Posture.   I. Worthingham,
  Catherine A., joint author.   II. Title.   [DNLM:
  1. Gymnastics. WB541 D187t]

RM725.D36 1977   616.7′4′0754   76–27058

ISBN 0–7216–2873–7

Therapeutic Exercise for Body Alignment and Function   ISBN   0-7216-2873-7

Last digit is the print number: 9   8   7   6   5   4   3   2   1

The Second Edition of Therapeutic Exercise is dedicated to Marian Williams, Ph.D., former co-author, distinguished colleague, and loyal friend.

PREFACE
TO THE SECOND EDITION

This textbook has been designed for the use of persons dealing with the problems of body alignment and function, primarily the physical therapist, the physical educator, and the physician. Those procedures are included that appear to be best suited for prevention of disability, improvement of impaired function, and maintenance of the optimum level of activity. The content is directed to the treatment of the ambulatory patient; however, the exercises may be adapted to various types of disability and to individuals at different age levels.

The material presented in the first edition was developed over a period of years for classes in corrective physical education and physical therapy by Dr. Worthingham and Dr. Marian Williams, co-authors of the first edition. Before publication, it had been made available to other schools for a number of years in mimeographed form, bound by the Stanford University Press.

The second edition has been completely revised in an attempt to provide a clearer and more concise teaching tool for students and an improved reference book for those in practice. The concern is with selection and analysis of basic material rather than with the introduction of new techniques. Since many of the procedures have been in general use, it would be impossible to acknowledge a source for each.

An appendix giving a brief review of the anatomical location and role of the primary muscles concerned with body alignment and function was included in the first edition. This appendix has been eliminated and pertinent anatomical information included throughout the text. The third edition of *Muscle Testing* by the same authors and publisher contains more extensive anatomical information. In addition, the test positions form a basis for exercises designed to increase the strength of specific muscles or muscle groups weakened from disuse, disease, or injury. This edition of *Therapeutic Exercise* has been designed as a companion text.

The authors are indebted to the many instructors in schools of physical therapy who have used the first edition over a period of years for their suggestions and to the members of the faculty of the Division of Physical Therapy at Stanford University for their contributions and support.

LUCILLE DANIELS

CATHERINE WORTHINGHAM

CONTENTS

I ANALYSIS AND EVALUATION OF BODY ALIGNMENT

The case for good body alignment as it relates to functional efficiency has been stated by many persons over the years. The subject has been approached from several aspects, including the physiological, the mechanical, the psychological, and the esthetic. Its importance as a preventive for those chronic disabilities developing from the stress and strain of occupations, fatigue, and the passing years is receiving new emphasis with the increasing attention to the geriatric population. In fact, interest in body alignment is not surprising, as it affects everyone regardless of activities, environment, or age.

Three major factors influence adult posture: inheritance, disease, and habit. Familial characteristics such as type of bone structure and variations in trunk and extremity proportion need to be identified and carefully considered in the approach to treatment. The effects of debilitating and deforming disease often require limitations on the type and amount of activity, and a careful gradation of exercise. Poor body alignment, whether from occupational demands or faulty postural habits, eventually limits normal function.

The approach to improved alignment and function by means of specific exercises is based on the concept that postural adjustment is a homeostatic mechanism which may be voluntarily controlled to a large degree. Repeated conscious correction of faulty alignment and maintenance of good position leads to improved habits. For example, a person with a mild spinal curvature may feel comfortable although he can see in a mirror that his trunk is deviated. When his position is corrected, he feels strange at first even though his eyes tell him he is now straight. He must constantly correct and overcorrect until he can recognize by proprioceptive means that he is in a good position and that the former unbalanced alignment now makes him feel uncomfortable.

Training of the person's kinesthetic sense is a fundamental factor in the correction of body alignment. It is especially important during the period of growth as the body tissues and organs are very responsive to stresses placed upon them.

THEORETICAL BACKGROUND FOR EVALUATION OF STANDING ALIGNMENT

The procedures for evaluation of the alignment of the individual which are basic to a plan for therapeutic exercise are presented in relation to the effect of gravity.

FORCE OF GRAVITY

The body is constantly subjected to the force of gravity in whatever position is assumed. This force is utilized to stabilize the lower extremities in standing and to provide the necessary friction for locomotion. At the same time it places considerable stress on the structures of the body that are responsible for maintenance of the upright position. Consequently, so-called postural deviations are common, and acute distress and disability affect large numbers of persons as a result of strain and injury to antigravity structures.

1

CENTER OF GRAVITY

The concept of the center of gravity of the body is basic to an analysis of any position of rest and movement, and therefore is a concept fundamental to all considerations of body alignment and function.

The center of gravity is a point at the exact center of the mass of the body. Its location varies among individuals according to their build. In a given subject, it also moves upward, downward, or sideward in accordance with changes in the position of the body segments during activity. Any object behaves as though its entire mass were centered at this point. Actually, the human body is made up of a number of movable segments, each of which has its own center. However, in a consideration of standing alignment the entire body may be visualized as a whole, with the height of the center of gravity in the region of the second sacral vertebra.

DETERMINATION OF THE CENTER OF GRAVITY

The importance of the location of this center of the body is reflected in the vast amount of attention it has received in the literature.

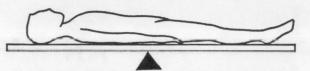

Figure 1. Early method for determining the height of the center of gravity of the body.

As early as the seventeenth century, Borelli originated the time-honored method of using a plank balanced over a wedge. The subject was placed supine on the plank and moved back and forth until balance was obtained (Fig. 1).

Over the years, others have determined by varying methods that the center of gravity lay between 55 and 57.99 per cent of the distance from the soles of the feet to the top of the head.

Variability in the location of the center according to age and sex was stressed by Meyer, Palmer, and Scheidt.

VISUALIZATION OF THE GRAVITY OR WEIGHT LINE

The gravity or weight line is the vertical projection of the center of gravity with the subject in the standing position. It may be visualized as an imaginary plumb line pass-

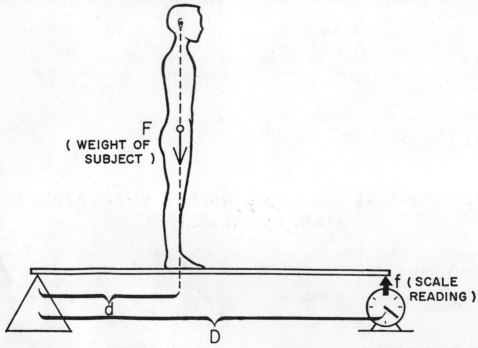

Figure 2. A convenient method for determining the position of the gravity line of the body (vertical projection from the center of gravity). The length of d can be computed by the formula $d \times F = D \times f$. F, f, and D can be measured; thus $d = \dfrac{D \times f}{F}$. This gives an accurate picture of anteroposterior balance. To find the gravity line in relation to lateral balance, the subject faces forward on the board.

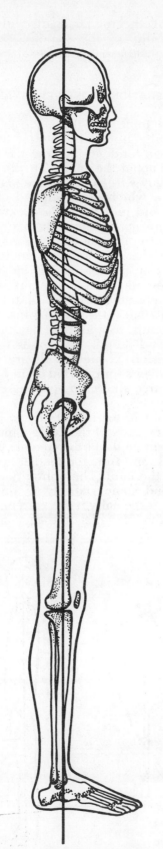

Figure 3. The vertical gravity line of the body.

ing through the center of gravity of the body.

The scale method, which has been widely used in research, provides a means of determining both the height of the center of gravity and the position of the gravity or weight line (Fig. 2).

The line has been described as falling midway between the heel and the heads of the metatarsals, slightly in front of the transverse axis of rotation at the knee joint, through or posterior to the hip joint, in front of the atlanto-occipital joint, and through the lobe of the ear (Fig. 3).

THE PHYSIOLOGICAL CURVES

In the embryo and newborn infant, the spine is flexed without the anteroposterior curves of the adult. The first lordotic curve takes place in the cervical region as the child extends his neck from the prone position. During the early development, on sitting upright and standing, the child's thoracic spine straightens and the lordotic curve in the lumbar region begins to appear. The curves in the cervical and lumbar areas become accentuated with growth according to the stress and strain of the antigravity positions.

In the adult, the cervical vertebrae, viewed laterally, form a symmetrical anterior convex curve, the thoracic vertebrae curve posteriorly, and the lumbar vertebrae reverse in the anterior direction—a total of three curves. It has been noted that there is

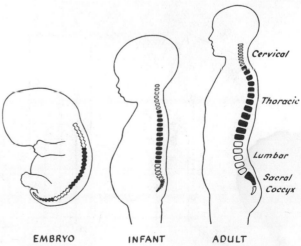

EMBRYO   INFANT   ADULT

Figure 4. Spinal contour at different age levels (from Jones, L.: The Postural Complex. Springfield, Ill., Charles C Thomas, 1955).

a sharp angulation above C1 (atlas) to allow the head to be on a level horizontal plane. This has been referred to as the fourth physiological curve.

STABILIZING MECHANISMS OF THE STANDING POSITION

MECHANICAL BALANCE

A weight-bearing joint will be mechanically balanced and in equilibrium only if the gravity line of the mass it supports falls exactly through the axis of rotation. If the line falls anterior to the axis, the upper part, or segment, tends to rotate in a forward direction. If it falls posterior to the axis, the upper segment tends to rotate backward. The vertical projection of the center of gravity of the body passes anterior to the axis of the knee and ankle joints; it is usually described as posterior to the axis of the hip joint. Consequently, in each case there is a tendency toward rotation of the upper segment about the axis of the supporting joints (Fig. 5).

FOOT PLACEMENT

For the standing position to be stable, the line of gravity must fall well within the base of support. The placement of the feet, whether parallel or in a toe-out position,

close together or far apart, will influence the stability of the standing position by providing a base of variable size (Fig. 6).

CONSIDERATION OF INDIVIDUAL JOINTS

Ankle Joint. At the ankle joint, where the gravity line falls anterior to the axis, there is a tendency for the tibia to rotate forward about the ankle. This is prevented by the guy-wire action of the plantar flexor muscles, which are anchored on the calcaneus and pull the tibia backward. Ligaments are not an element in support here because the limit of the joint range has not been reached. Therefore, standing balance requires a degree of muscular activity. Considerable passive support is afforded by the elastic properties of the two-joint gastrocnemius muscle. Wearing shoes with heels tends to put this muscle "on the slack" and thereby decreases the supportive tension. If high heels are worn constantly over a long period of time there may be adaptive shortening of the Achilles tendon muscles.

Another factor in stability to be considered is the axis of the ankle joint. This lies at a slight angle to the frontal plane, passing backward from the medial to the lateral side of the joint. The obliquity of this axis may lend some stability to the standing posture, especially if the extremities are in a position in which the feet are pointed

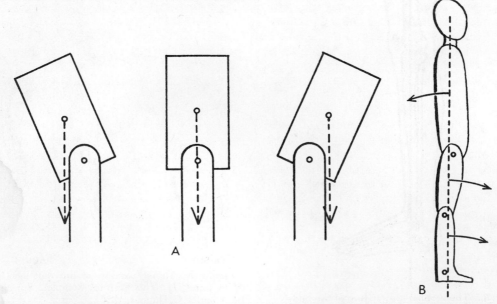

Figure 5. *A,* Balance is achieved only in the center figure. *B,* In normal relaxed standing, the leg, thigh, and trunk all tend to rotate either forward or backward away from the midline.

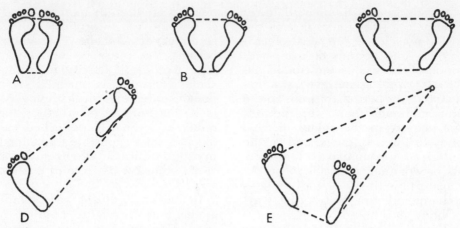

Figure 6. Various foot positions in standing which provide varying areas of support. The base increases in size from *A* to *D*. *E* illustrates the large area of support made possible by the use of a cane. Crutches would increase the base considerably.

slightly outward, as the plane of flexion of the joints is at an angle to the anteroposterior plane in which the body tends to sway forward and backward. A person with weak plantar flexor muscles may maintain equilibrium by keeping his weight farther back than normal and balanced directly over the ankle joints.

Knee Joint. At the knee joint the weight line in standing is again anterior to the axis. Here, however, forward rotation of the femur on the tibia is prevented by the strong posterior, collateral, and cruciate ligaments, as well as by the muscles passing over the posterior aspect of the joint. Activity of the knee extensor muscles is not required. Therefore, a person with weak quadriceps femoris muscles has no difficulty in standing as long as he keeps his knees fully extended and his center of gravity well forward. Smith has argued that the hamstrings rather than the knee extensors are situated as prime movers to resist the force of gravity at this joint.

Meyer believed that when tension is placed on the iliofemoral ligament in full hip extension, the oblique direction of the ligamentous fibers causes internal rotation of the femur, which contributes to the locking of the knee. Tension of the iliofemoral band was also said to prevent knee flexion so that no quadriceps femoris action is necessary for support.

Another feature in the stability of the knee joint is the thigh rotation or "screw home" mechanism accompanying the final phase of complete extension. In this movement, the femur rides backward on its medial condyle and rotates medially about its vertical axis to "lock" the joint for weight bearing. At the beginning of knee flexion this process is reversed, and the femur is rotated laterally in relation to the tibia.

Hip Joint. At the hip joint the weight line usually passes posterior to the joint axis. Consequently, the tendency of the trunk is to fall backward. Here we are concerned with the center of gravity of the suprafemoral mass which is balanced over the hip joints. According to duBois-Reymond, the center of gravity of the trunk, head, and arms combined lies 0.86 cm. posterior to the hip axis. On the other hand, Meyer placed it 5 cm. behind the hip axis. It is probable that this distance varies considerably from person to person according to body build and habitual posture. Posterior rotation of the trunk is prevented by the structures that cross the anterior aspect of the hip joint, principally the iliofemoral ligament and the hip flexor muscles.

Kelton and Wright concluded from anatomic studies that the fascia lata is significant in lateral stabilization but not in hyperextension at the hip. No mention was made of its function of bracing the knee when it is fully extended. These authors described a so-called easy standing position, in which stability is brought about by muscle action. In this position the feet are separated by approximately the interacetabular distance, and the extremities are externally rotated about 25 degrees.

ACTION POTENTIALS IN MUSCLES

With the subject in the position just described, the same authors recorded muscle action potentials from a number of lower extremity muscles. They found that all the thigh and leg muscles tested were electrically silent for long periods of time, with the exception of the soleus and tibialis anterior. These were sometimes simultaneously inactive for periods of from one to five seconds, although there were periods of constant activity in the soleus of from five seconds to three minutes, and in the tibialis anterior of from two to forty seconds. This predominance of activity in the soleus as against the tibialis anterior relates to the predominantly anteroposterior swaying of the body, as studied by other investigators, in which it was found that the weight was almost always in front of the axis of the ankle and knee joints and posterior to the axis of the hip.

Other investigators, utilizing the electromyograph, have likewise demonstrated that surprisingly little active muscle contraction is used to maintain the standing position. Joseph and Nightingale found activity in the calf muscles, particularly the soleus, but electrical silence in the tibialis anterior. Hoefer found very little activity in either the gastrocnemius or tibialis anterior in seven standing subjects. He concluded that the elastic properties of muscle may maintain posture. Floyd and Silver found very little electrical activity when standing in an easy position, but that very small deviations from this position called forth spurts of flexor and extensor activity.

After reviewing electromyographic evidence Ralston and Libet ask, "What does maintain a sitting or standing posture if not relatively continuous active muscle contraction serving to lock the joints in position?" They agree that balancing of the body parts and tension resulting from passive stretch of fascial sheets, ligaments, and muscles are primary factors which act before muscle action is called into play. It is possible that differences in the so-called "easy standing position" utilized by the different investigators account for the slight variation in their results.

The intermittent nature of muscle contraction that has been observed in standing is closely associated with the question of neurologic control of this position. Control is generally recognized as an automatic process, which Hellebrandt has termed a "geotropic reflex." According to the concept of Sherrington, shifts in position at the joints may cause stretching of the antigravity muscles; tonic contractions of these muscles are thereby increased and the joint is restored to its original position. More recent experiments have raised doubts concerning the presence of constant active tone (motor unit activity) in normal, resting skeletal muscle, as repeated sampling has demonstrated electrical silence. Also, there is a question as to whether the stretch reflex as ordinarily described can be the mechanism responsible for maintaining the upright position when such extremely slight adjustments in joint position are involved.

In summary, during easy standing there appear to be intermittent periods of activity in the appropriate antigravity muscles which restore the upright position accompanied by a constant slight swaying of the body.

OSCILLATION OF THE BODY IN STANCE

Smith has pointed out that there are two types of oscillation when the subject is standing at ease: the slower and larger in a backward and forward movement, the smaller in a series of oscillations to and fro. Bowman and Jalavisto reported the anteroposterior magnitude of these oscillations in 45 subjects between 18 and 30 years of age was 41.7 ± 1.6 mm., and the lateral sway 29.7 ± 8 mm. Hellebrandt and co-workers, in a series of studies, investigated the nature and magnitude of body sway. It was found to be largely anteroposterior in direction, and was repeated in a fairly constant pattern which was remarkably characteristic for each person. The average area of maximal sway for a group of men and women was found to be approximately 4 cm. The mean vertical projection of the center of gravity was slightly behind and to the left of the center of the base of support in standing.

There seems to be general agreement that the extent of the swaying in the "standing at ease position" is such that the weight is almost always in front of the ankle joint, usually in front of the knee joints, and normally in front of the axis of the hips, so that there is a tendency to fall forward.

Effect of Prolonged Stance

Smith has investigated the attitudes of standing assumed during prolonged stance.

Two hundred and fifty subjects were observed for at least two minutes, none knowing he was under observation. Two basic positions were observed: 1) a symmetrical stance with the weight distributed equally on both feet, and 2) an asymmetrical stance, in which nearly all the weight rests on one foot. The asymmetrical attitude occurred about four times as often as the symmetrical. The mean duration of all positions was about 30 seconds, and 93 per cent were maintained for less than one minute. Frequent shifting of position allows brief periods of rest to the supporting tissues of the body during long immobile standing. Alternation between asymmetrical weight bearing on the right and left foot extends the rest periods and renders intermittent the pressure effects of gravity. In Smith's opinion, habitual prolongation of the immobile periods, such as might be required in certain types of work, may lead to postural disorders.

ALERT AND RELAXED STANCE

Among others, Mommsen has differentiated between "alert" and "relaxed" standing positions. When a person is under tension in standing (for example, when he tries to appear as erect as possible), the trunk weight may be exactly balanced over the hip joints in the sagittal plane. However, in ordinary "relaxed" standing, particularly over a long period of time, it is more common for the pelvis to shift slightly forward and the upper trunk backward, so that the gravity line of the trunk falls well behind the hip axis. Other terms that have been used to describe the quality of the standing posture are "comfortable position" and "military position."

SUMMARY OF THEORETICAL BACKGROUND

Standing posture involves a welding of the various segments of the body into a mechanically stable whole. The skeletal parts are supported over the feet by the "passive" tension of ligaments, by the fascia, and by the elastic properties of muscle, as well as by a minimal amount of "active" contraction of motor units in certain stabilizing muscles. In relaxed symmetrical standing, both the hip and the knee joints assume a position of full extension as they support the superincumbent weight. The knee joint has an additional stabilizing element in its "screw home" mechanism: here, rotation is superimposed on full extension to lock the joint more firmly. At the ankle joint there is no bony or ligamentous limit to motion; however, passive tension of the two-joint gastrocnemius muscle is a factor in stability, since the knee is extended and the body leans slightly forward from the ankles. This stabilizing force is decreased by the wearing of high-heeled shoes. It is not surprising that in standing action potentials are present primarily in those muscles that act around the ankle joint. Body sway accompanying the normal relaxed upright position is limited by intermittent activity to appropriate antigravity muscles, which are under automatic control. In prolonged standing the average person shifts his position frequently, assuming both symmetrical and asymmetrical attitudes but primarily the latter.

With this brief introduction we turn to specific procedures in the evaluation of body alignment. It will be evident that many of the so-called postural deviations observed in the standing subject are exaggerations of the normal stabilizing mechanisms; examples are hyperextended knees, lordosis, and extreme out-toe positions of the feet.

EVALUATION OF STANDING ALIGNMENT

An appraisal of body alignment serves three principal objectives: the results serve as a guide for the exercise program; they provide a record for future reference from which to evaluate progress; and they give the person examined a concept of his body alignment. At the same time, the examiner has the opportunity to obtain information concerning other factors about the person that may be contributing to poor alignment, such as malnutrition, fatigue, hypertonicity, and psychological states.

A number of procedures have been described in which specific grading is based on reasonably definite criteria in order to judge alignment as accurately as possible. Among others, Cureton and Clarke have summarized the available methods.

Many workers investigating body alignment have made use of mechanical aids in an attempt to increase the objectivity of measurement. There is a danger, however, that the beginner may become so preoccupied with slight deviations of the various segments that he may miss the more basic picture of overall body balance. For this reason it is advised that the student first master the method of sighting total alignment and then estimating deviations with a grade of "slight," "moderate," or "extreme" degree. After he has grasped the fundamental concept of "good" and "poor" alignment of the body segments and has gained proficiency in judging alignment by inspection, he may then wish to use such apparatus as goniometers, metal pointers, and spirit levels in a further refinement of his techniques.

The various points to be recorded in the examination of body alignment are indicated in the record form (page 11). It is suggested that *extreme deviation* in alignment or function *be recorded in red* to focus attention quickly on areas requiring particular consideration.

Appraisal of deviations in alignment, like other specific conditions of the body, rests on the concept of a so-called "normal" standard. This standard is the "idealistic" or "perfect" concept, which is seldom if ever attained. The examiner should keep in mind that individuals differ in body type and, because of this fact, may be expected to vary in acceptable postural alignment.

BODY TYPE

Differences in body type, and the characteristics that go with them, have been recognized and studied by many persons. Sheldon and later Cureton made particularly valuable contributions in this area.

Sheldon divided people into three major types, endomorphic, mesomorphic and ectomorphic. The endomorphic type he characterized as round, soft, and smooth in contour, with a predominance of abdomen over thorax, high squared shoulders, and short neck. He described the mesomorphic type as having large bones covered with thick muscle. The thorax is large, the waist comparatively slender, the abdominal muscles prominent and thick. He depicted the ectomorphic type as more linear and fragile, with small bones and thin muscles; the shoulders droop and the scapulae tend to wing.

From a photographic analysis of 4000 males, Sheldon determined that the pure types do not exist, that each individual has some traces of all three elements. He developed a scaling technique based on five regions for the three components; the technique is quite elaborate and too expensive for general use.

Some years later Cureton developed a more simplified method for determining the somatotype based on Sheldon's work. The method, which is rated on a scale of one to seven, considers external fat, muscular development and condition, and skeletal development.

For purposes of the postural evaluation here described, an estimate of body type as "lithe," "medium," or "stout" provides some indication of these factors as determinants of body alignment. Judgment may be utilized in selecting the predominant type or overlapping types by describing them as "medium lithe" or "medium stout."

BODY ALIGNMENT

The first step in evaluating standing posture is to sight the overall balance of the body. An attempt should be made to have the person at ease, to avoid rigid and unnatural positions. The subject's body weight (anteroposterior balance) should be evenly supported and not shifted far forward over the balls of the feet, or backward over the heels (Fig. 7). Similarly, the individual's weight (lateral balance) should be borne evenly on both feet and not shifted to either the right or left sides predominantly (Fig. 8).

The deviations from the gravity lines are from the stable point, the contact with the floor, as the standing position involves a series of superincumbent segments, all of which are balanced over the feet.

It is helpful when judging alignment to suspend a plumb line by hand, sited at a point just anterior to the lateral malleolus for anteroposterior deviations and midway between the heels for lateral deviations. A grid on a wall behind the subject can also provide a constant background for this purpose.

Caution should be used in grading seg-mental deviations in relation to their neighboring segments. This procedure is valid *only* if the segment used for reference is in good position, which is often not the case.

Because the person may tend to correct his specific faults momentarily even though he is unaware of doing so, it is important to glance back from time to time to make sure his position has not changed significantly.

When the student has developed the ability to check body alignment by the teaching sequence suggested on page 11, a consolidated record sheet may be utilized, using symbols for recording (page 22). This record requires less space, is easier to read at a glance, and has the advantage of easy conversion to a computer record.

Both the Analysis of Limited Activities (page 24) and the Analysis of Basic Activities (page 34) can be placed on the back of either record form.

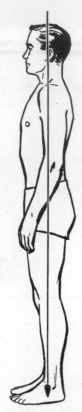

Figure 7. Anteroposterior gravity line.

EVALUATION OF STANDING ALIGNMENT

ANTEROPOSTERIOR GRAVITY LINE

Passes through:
1. head — ear lobe
2. shoulder — center of tip
3. hip — greater trochanter of femur
4. knee — posterior to the patella
5. foot — anterior to the lateral malleolus of the fibula

Individuals having an abnormal degree of mobility tend to exaggerate spinal curves and to stand with the hip and knee joints hyperextended. The pelvis is tilted forward, the thorax backward, and the head forward. The distance from the hip and knee axes to the vertical line is greater than normal.

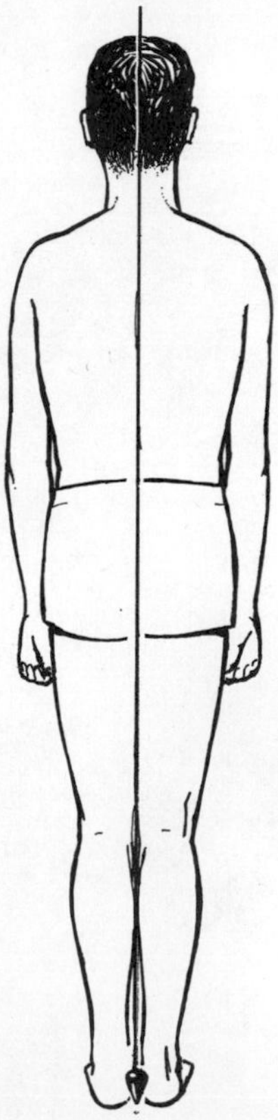

Figure 8. Lateral gravity line.

LATERAL GRAVITY LINE

Passes through:
1. head — occipital protuberance
2. spine — spinous process of 7th cervical vertebra
3. hips — cleft of the buttocks
4. knees — space midway between medial borders
5. feet — space midway between heels

Judged from the posterior or anterior view, the gravity line ideally bisects the body into two symmetrical halves. Although slight deviations are common, irregularities in symmetry beyond a minor degree should be carefully noted. For lateral spinal deviations, see Scoliosis, pages 15–17.

Evaluation of Standing Alignment

Name _____ Birth Date _____

Body Type   Lithe (   )   Medium (   )   Stout (   )
                    Medium Lithe (   )   Medium Stout (   )

Pain: If present, note as Slight, Moderate, or Extreme in Remarks column				
Date				Specific information or remarks with dates
*Body Alignment	Grade:	Grade:	Grade:	
Lateral View				
Body displaced anteriorly				
Body displaced posteriorly				
Head forward				
Scapulae projected				
Thoracic curve increased (kyphosis)				
Lumbar curve increased (lordosis)				
Abdomen protruded				
Knees hyperextended				
Longitudinal arch of foot low				
Other				
Posterior View				
Body displaced laterally				
Head tilted laterally				
Scapulae abducted				
Waist angles uneven				
Spine curved laterally (scoliosis)				
Back flat				
Feet pronated				
Other				
Anterior View				
Shoulder high				
Rib cage abnormal				
Pelvic level uneven				
Legs misaligned				
Toes misaligned**				
Other				
Overall alignment: Good Fair Poor				

*Key to Grading—No deviation:− Slight: 1 Moderate: 2 Extreme: 3 Right: R Left: L
**Use I–V for toe identification

EVALUATION OF STANDING ALIGNMENT

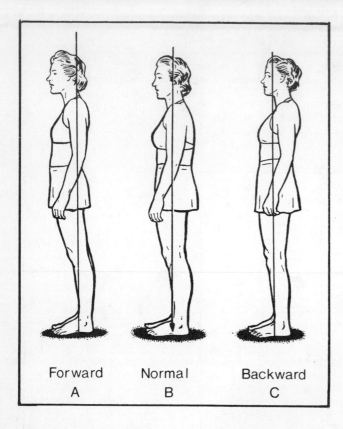

Forward
A

Normal
B

Backward
C

LATERAL VIEW

ANTEROPOSTERIOR BALANCE

Forward or backward shifting of the body weight should not be confused with the natural tendency of the body to sway during standing. It should be rechecked during the examination and entered in the record only if a deviation is definitely characteristic of the subject's stance.

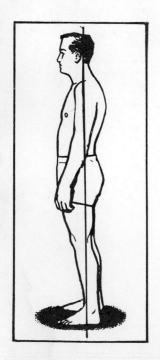

HEAD

Forward head is judged in relation to the vertical gravity line of the body in which the lobe of the ear should be directly over the tip of the shoulder. However, if, as in the illustration, the acromion is not on that line because the scapulae are tipped forward, the judgment of head position should be made in relation to the line, not the acromion.

EVALUATION OF STANDING ALIGNMENT

LATERAL VIEW

SCAPULAE

Projection is a prominence of the inferior angle of the scapulae, or, in some cases, of the entire vertebral border. It is the result of rotation or a tilting forward of the scapulae, or both.

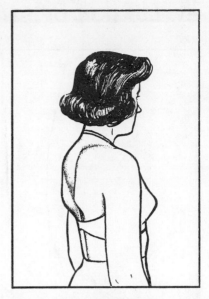

SPINE

Kyphosis is an increase of the normal posteriorly convex thoracic curve (illustrated).

Lordosis is an exaggeration of the normal anteriorly concave lumbar curve (not illustrated).

Kypholordosis is a combination of the two deviations described above in which each is severe (not illustrated).

Round back is a rounding of the greater extent of the spine in a posterior direction. There may be a sharp angle at the base of the spine or lower lumbar area and an anterior tilt of the pelvis. In other instances the pelvis may be in a neutral or posteriorly rotated position (not illustrated).

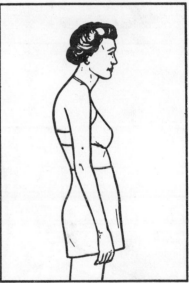

ABDOMEN

Relaxation or weakness of the abdominal muscles results in protrusion of the abdominal wall.

Note: Young children have a natural prominence of the abdominal wall. Women may have a deposit of fat lying transversely across the abdomen, just below the umbilicus and external to the muscle layer, which can confuse the examiner by making the protrusion more apparent than real.

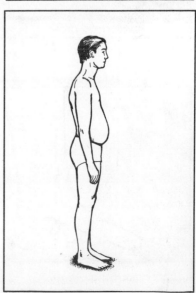

EVALUATION OF STANDING ALIGNMENT

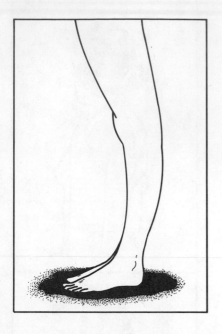

LATERAL VIEW

LEGS

Knees are hyperextended (genu recurvatum) if the line of the femur forms an anterior obtuse angle with the line of the tibia. In all leg alignment tests, the examiner should visualize the bony skeleton and not be misled by the muscle contours. Recheck to see if the position recorded is habitual.

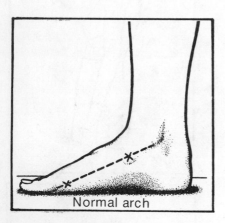

Normal arch

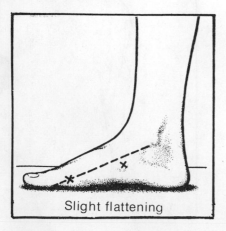

Slight flattening

LONGITUDINAL ARCH

Depression or flattening of the long arch of the foot is determined by the position of the navicular tubercle relative to a hypothetical line that extends from just below the medial malleolus to the point where the metatarsophalangeal joint of the great toe rests on the floor (Feiss' line). The space between the line and the floor may be divided into thirds for purposes of grading. Normally, the navicular tubercle is on the line. If it is one third of the distance to the floor it is recorded as slight (1), two thirds of the distance as moderate (2), and resting on the floor as extreme (3). A convex medial border of the foot is found in extreme flattening of the arch.

EVALUATION OF STANDING ALIGNMENT

POSTERIOR VIEW

LATERAL DISPLACEMENT OF BODY

A plumb line falling midway between the heels bisects the cleft of the buttocks, sacrum, seventh cervical, and occipital protuberance. In this illustration, there is lateral imbalance to the left. If posterior superior spines of the ilium are not level, leg lengths may not be equal and should be measured (not illustrated, see page 36).

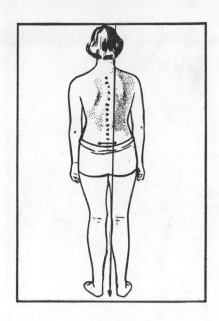

HEAD

A right head tilt means that the top of the head has moved to the right and the chin to the left. Visualize a horizontal line between the lobes of the ears and judge if it forms right angles to a vertical plumb line (not illustrated).

SCAPULAE

Scapular abduction is graded by the distance from the vertebral borders to the spinal column. The size and body type of the individual are considered. In the adult, approximately two inches would be recorded as slight (1), three inches as moderate (2), and four inches as extreme (3) (see illustration below).

WAIST ANGLES

The right or left waist angle may be more acute. A difference indicates a scoliotic asymmetry of the spine (see illustration page 17).

SPINE

Lateral Deviation of Spine

To determine the amount of lateral spinal deviation in a single (C) or a double (thoracolumbar) curve if scoliosis is present, locate the center of the trunk by stretching a plumb line from the spinous process of the seventh cervical vertebra to the center of the lumbosacral junction (illustrated). Measure the distance between the apex of the curve or curves and the plumb line. For a cervical curve, stretch the plumb line between the center of the occipital line of the head and the seventh cervical and use the same procedure.

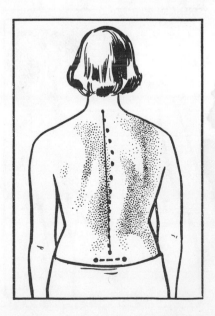

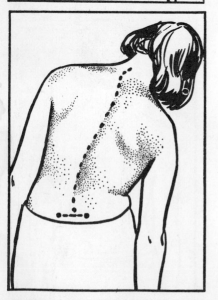

POSTERIOR VIEW

SPINE

Structural Scoliosis

Have the subject flex the trunk laterally. In the structural curve illustrated, the right thoracic curve is free when the trunk is flexed toward its concavity (left), but remains rigid during flexion toward the convexity (right). The mild left curve is freer but has more limitation in flexion to the left than to the right. The thoracic curve has undergone greater structural change and is thus termed the "primary" curve, the lumbar the "secondary."

EVALUATION OF STANDING ALIGNMENT

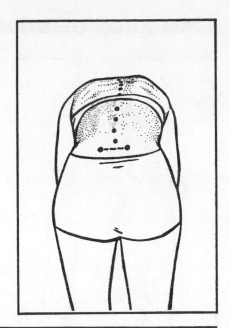

Ask the subject to lean forward, head and arms dropped in a relaxed manner. The curves disappear if structural changes have not taken place. In the illustration, structural rotation is evidenced by the prominence on the convexity of the curve.

Grade the severity of curves, record the measurements of the amount of spinal deviation, and identify primary and secondary curves under Remarks.

Measure leg lengths (page 36). Look for asymmetry in leg alignment, such as unilateral knock knee, tibial torsion, flat foot, or extreme out-toe position of one foot.

Cross Section of Trunk

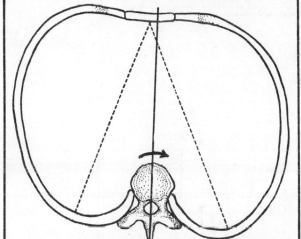

A cross section diagram in the region of the midthorax may help to clarify the external configuration of the trunk. In a right thoracic curve, the heads of the ribs are pulled backward on the right, and the anterior rib extremities are prominent on the left.

Postural Scoliosis

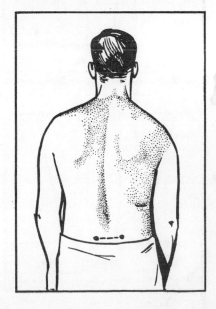

The left total curve (C curve) illustrated is typical of a postural scoliosis. A mild degree of vertebral rotation is evidenced by asymmetry of the posterior thorax on the right and left sides. The left shoulder is high, with scapular abduction and slight projection. A skin crease is present on the concave side of the waist line. This type of scoliosis disappears when the trunk is flexed in the standing position (see structural scoliosis).

Grade curve and identify as R or L postural under Remarks.

EVALUATION OF STANDING ALIGNMENT

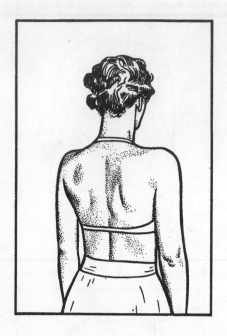

POSTERIOR VIEW

SPINE

Flat back is a decrease or absence of the normal anteroposterior spinal curves.

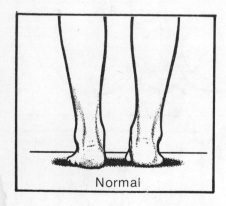

Normal

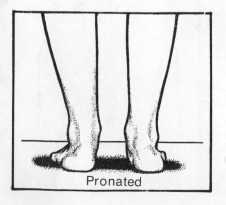

Pronated

FEET

In foot pronation, the line of the Achilles tendon slants medialward. This deviation involves eversion of the calcaneus, which takes place primarily at the subtalar articulation and should not be termed *ankle* pronation. While pes planus, or flat foot, is commonly associated with foot pronation, the two are different deviations.

EVALUATION OF STANDING ALIGNMENT

ANTERIOR VIEW

SHOULDERS

Left high or right high is recorded only when there is a definite difference in the height of the scapulae as judged by position of the clavicles. Judgment is assisted by the use of a horizontal line on the wall behind the subject.

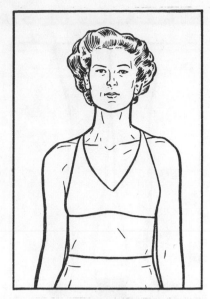

CHEST

Hollow chest, or a flattened appearance of the anterior thoracic wall (sternum and ribs depressed and lowered), is commonly associated with an increased anteroposterior thoracic spinal curve. Other deviations involving structural changes (not illustrated) are funnel, barrel, and pigeon chest.

Harrison's groove (illustrated) is a transverse depression across the lower region of the thorax. The ribs may flare out distal to the groove. A transverse groove frequently present in the soft tissue just below the thorax should not be mistaken for a true bony deformity involving structural changes in the ribs.

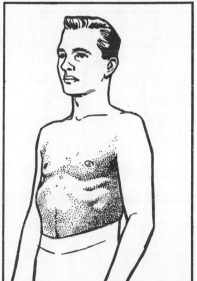

PELVIS

Determination of the pelvic level may be made from the relative heights of the anterior superior iliac spines. A tape stretched between these points may be helpful in sighting alignment. Further comparison of levels can be made by fitting the hands (with palms down) over the two iliac crests.

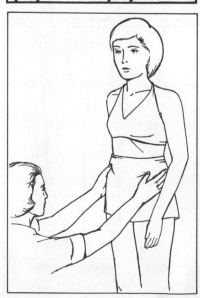

EVALUATION OF STANDING ALIGNMENT

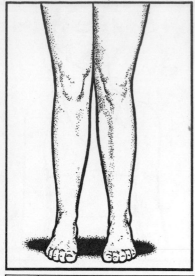

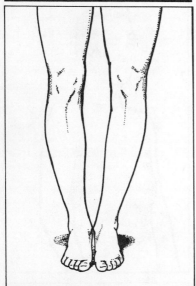

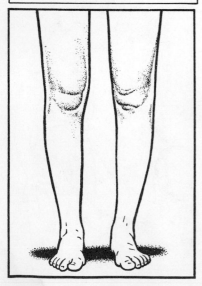

ANTERIOR VIEW

LEGS

Knock knees (genu valgum) are judged by having the person stand with the patellae facing straight ahead and the medial border of the knees just touching. If there are more than a few centimeters of space between the medial malleoli, genu valgum is present. It may be more marked on one side than the other. This serves to shorten one leg and cause imbalance of the pelvis.

Bow legs (genu varum) are graded by having the subject stand with the medial malleoli just touching. The space between the knees determines the degree of genu varum. A distinction can be made between "functional" genu varum and true malalignment of the extremity in which the femur and tibia form a definite angle. Many flexible persons can push their knees back into hyperextension, which is associated with femoral rotation and genu varum. A skeletal deformity should be recorded only if it is present when the knees are comfortably extended but not forced back into full hyperextension.

Tibial torsion is estimated according to the position of the patellae with reference to the feet. The person stands with his feet parallel and slightly apart. If the patellae appear to be rolled inward in a "cross-eyed" position, tibial torsion is recorded (illustrated). Or, if the subject stands with the patellae straight ahead, his feet point outward, showing lateral rotation of the tibia on the femur. This deviation is often more marked in one extremity than the other.

EVALUATION OF STANDING ALIGNMENT

ANTERIOR VIEW

TOES

Hallux valgus is a marked deviation of the great toe toward the midline of the foot. This adduction at the metatarsophalangeal joint is sometimes associated with a bunion or callus on the medial border of the foot near the metatarsophalangeal joint. Deviation of the distal phalanx of the hallux at the interphalangeal joint should not be mistaken for true hallux valgus.

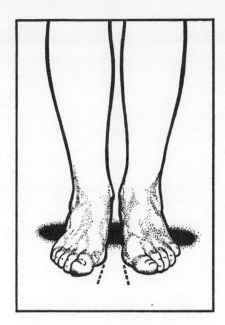

Hammer toes are recorded with the numbers of the digits involved. In this deviation the toe is sharply hyperextended at the metatarsophalangeal joint and flexed distally, as though the digit had buckled as a result of pressure against the end of the toe. Both the long flexor and extensor muscles may be shortened, and corns or calluses may have formed on the dorsal surfaces of the affected toes due to the pressure of shoes.

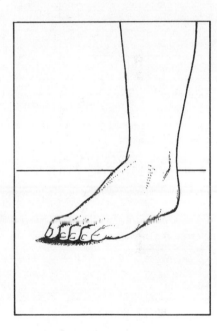

Record of Standing Alignment

Name_____Birth Date_____

Body type	Lithe ( )	Medium ( )	Stout ( )	Medium Lithe ( )	Medium Stout ( )
Date					Remarks
Presence of pain					
Anteroposterior balance					
Lateral balance					
Head					
Chest					
Shoulder level					
Scapulae					
Pelvic level					
Abdomen					
Spine					
Legs					
Foot — Pronation					
Long arch					
Metatarsal area					
Toes					
Overall Alignment					

Key
- − normal
- 1 slight
- 2 moderate
- 3 extreme
- R right
- L left

Body type
- L lithe
- M medium
- S stout

Anteroposterior
balance
- F forward
- B backward

Head
- F forward
- T tilt

Shoulders
- H high

Scapulae
- S separation
- P projection

Spine
- K kyphosis
- L lordosis
- R round
- F flat
- S scoliosis
  - P postural or functional
  - St structural
    - C cervical
    - T thoracic
    - L lumbar

Abdomen
- R relaxed

Legs
- KK knock knees
- BL bow legs
- H hyperextended knees
- TT tibial torsion

Feet
- P foot pronation
- F flat
- C callus metatarsal heads I–V

Toes
- HV hallux valgus I–V
- HT hammer toes I–V

Overall alignment
- G good
- F fair
- P poor

FOR NOTES:

EVALUATION OF LIMITED MOTION

Certain muscles and muscle groups frequently are found to be shortened in individuals with poor alignment. A primary causative factor may be an adaptive change in length brought about by habitual position or muscle usage. Tight muscles resist effort to assume a better position. If the examiner suspects shortening in additional groups, these also should be checked.

Illustrations and brief discussion of muscle functions are correlated with suggested tests for tightness to facilitate understanding. More detailed anatomical information and tests of muscle function will be found in the text *Muscle Testing*.

Evaluation of Limited Motion
(for muscles frequently shortened)

Name _____ Birth Date_____

Date					Remarks with date
Spine extensors					
Shoulder adductors and medial rotators					
Hip — flexors					
— abductors					
— adductors					
— lateral rotators					
Knee flexors					
Ankle plantar flexors					
Other					

Key
  — normal   limited: 1 slight
  R right   2 moderate
  L left   3 extreme

Note: Goniometric measurements may be recorded when motion is limited.

EVALUATION OF LIMITED MOTION

Extensors of Spine

Erector Spinae

Origin: Common tendon from posterior iliac crest, spinous processes of lower thoracic and lumbar vertebrae, and posterior aspect of sacrum. The muscle group forms three vertical columns: the *iliocostalis, longissimus* and *spinalis.*

Insertion: Spinous and transverse processes of cervical and thoracic vertebrae and adjacent area of ribs, mastoid process, and nuchal lines of the occipital bone. (Cervical and capitate portions are not illustrated.)

Semispinalis Cervicis

Origin: Transverse processes of upper five or six thoracic vertebrae.

Insertion: Spinous processes of second to fifth cervical vertebrae.

Splenius Capitis and Cervicis

Origin: Lower half of ligamentum nuchae, spinous processes of third through seventh cervical vertebrae and upper thoracic vertebrae.

Insertion: Mastoid process of adjacent area on occipital bone and transverse processes of upper two or three cervical vertebrae.

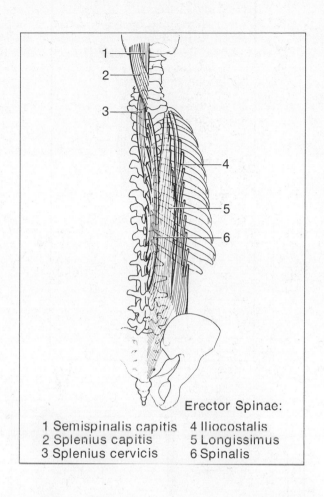

Erector Spinae:

1 Semispinalis capitis 4 Iliocostalis
2 Splenius capitis 5 Longissimus
3 Splenius cervicis 6 Spinalis

TEST FOR EXTENSORS OF THE SPINE

Flex neck and trunk from the supine position, arms at sides. Normally the lumbar and cervical spine straighten and the thoracic spine rounds.

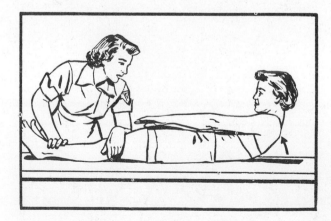

Alternate Test (if anterior hip, trunk or neck flexors are weak)

Sit on chair, knees apart. Flex hips, trunk, and neck until head and shoulders are between knees. Examiner stands in front to check range and stabilize knees if subject appears insecure.

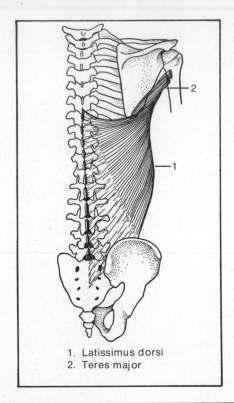

1. Latissimus dorsi
2. Teres major

SHOULDER ADDUCTORS AND MEDIAL ROTATORS

Latissimus Dorsi

Origin: Spinous processes of lower six thoracic vertebrae, spinous processes of lumbar and sacral vertebrae via lumbo-dorsal fascia, posterior crest of ilium, and lower three or four ribs.

Insertion: Bottom of intertubercular groove of humerus.

Teres Major

Origin: Dorsal surface of inferior angle of scapula.

Insertion: Crest below lesser tuberosity of humerus.

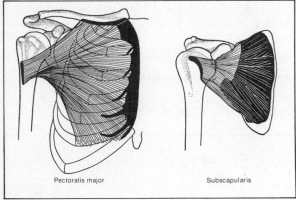

Pectoralis major   Subscapularis

Pectoralis Major

Origin: Sternal half of clavicle, ventral surface of sternum, and cartilages of first six or seven ribs.

Insertion: Crest of greater tubercle of humerus.

Subscapularis

Origin: Medial two thirds costal surface of scapula and inferior two thirds axillary border of scapula.

Insertion: Lesser tubercle of humerus.

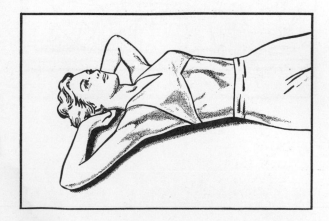

TEST FOR SHOULDER ADDUCTORS AND MEDIAL ROTATORS

The subject lies supine and places hands behind neck. With the lumbar spine as flat as possible, the elbows should rest on the table without strain. (Round back or kyphosis will prevent the completion of this test.) The knees may be flexed slightly to flatten the lumbar spine. Too much flexion will decrease tension of the abdominal muscles and remove their stabilizing action on the thorax.

FLEXORS OF HIP

Psoas Major

Origin: Sides of bodies of last thoracic and all lumbar vertebrae, intervertebral fibrocartilages, and transverse processes of all lumbar vertebrae.

Insertion: Lesser trochanter of femur.

Iliacus

Origin: Superior two thirds of iliac fossa, inner lip of iliac crest, and base of sacrum.

Insertion: Body of femur distal to lesser trochanter and lateral side of tendon of psoas major.

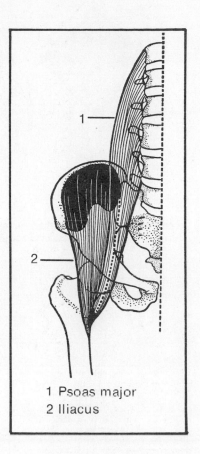

1 Psoas major
2 Iliacus

TEST FOR FLEXORS OF THE HIP

In the supine position, the subject pulls one thigh up against his chest, thereby posteriorly rotating the pelvis. If the hip flexors of the opposite extremity are not tight, the knee of the extended leg will remain on the table. Shortened hip flexors will cause the thigh to be lifted so that the knee is flexed (Thomas test).

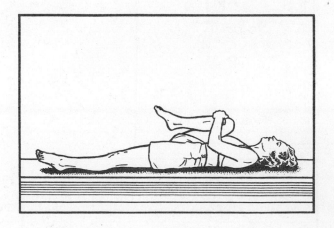

EVALUATION OF LIMITED MOTION

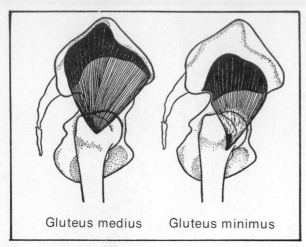

Gluteus medius   Gluteus minimus

ABDUCTORS OF THE HIP

Gluteus medius

Origin: Outer surface of ilium between anterior and posterior gluteal lines.

Insertion: Lateral surface of greater trochanter of femur.

Gluteus Minimus

Origin: Outer surface of ilium between anterior and inferior gluteal lines.

Insertion: Anterior surface of greater trochanter of femur.

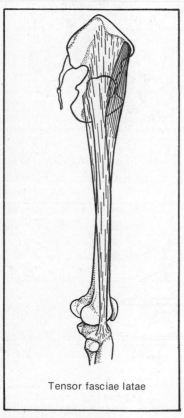

Tensor fasciae latae

Tensor Fasciae Latae

Origin: Anterior part of outer lip of iliac crest, outer surface superior iliac spine and notch below, and deep surface of fasciae latae.

Insertion: Iliotibial band at juncture of middle and upper thirds of the thigh.

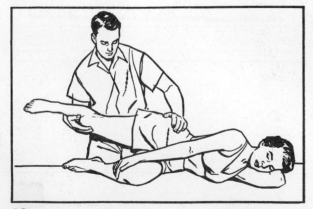

TEST FOR ABDUCTORS OF THE HIP

The subject lies on one side, holding the lower leg in flexion at the hip and knee. With one hand the examiner stabilizes the pelvis; with the other, he extends and adducts the thigh of the upper leg, holding the knee in flexion. If tightness is present in the abductors or iliotibial band, the thigh cannot be adducted to the midline of the body. The pelvis should not be allowed to rotate or tip laterally. (Based on the Ober test.)

ADDUCTORS OF THE HIP

Adductor Magnus, Adductor Brevis, Adductor Longus, Pectineus, and Gracilis

Origin: Superior and inferior rami of pubis and inferior ramus of ischium.

Insertion: Region of linea aspera and medial supracondylar line of femur. The gracilis crosses the knee to insert on the proximal end of the tibia.

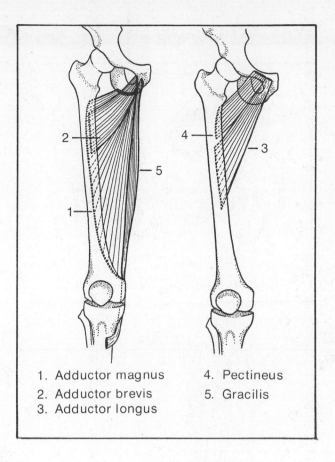

1. Adductor magnus
2. Adductor brevis
3. Adductor longus
4. Pectineus
5. Gracilis

TEST FOR ADDUCTORS OF THE HIP

Sidelying, with extremity underneath flexed for balance, the individual should be able to abduct the upper extremity to approximately 45 degrees. The thigh and trunk should not be rotated during the movement.

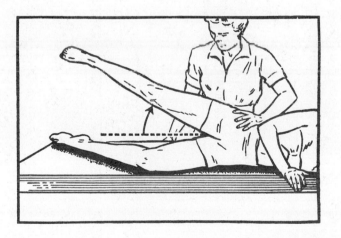

EVALUATION OF LIMITED MOTION

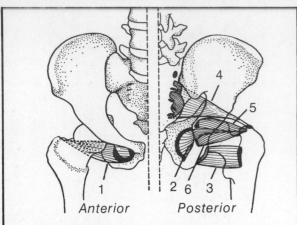

Anterior   *Posterior*

1. Obturator externus   4. Piriformis
2. Obturator internus   5. Gemellus superior
3. Quadratus femoris   6. Gemellus inferior

LATERAL ROTATORS OF THE HIP

Obturator Externus and Internus, Quadriceps Femoris, Piriformis, Gemellus Superior and Inferior, and Gluteus Maximus

Origin: Seven muscles are prime movers in hip lateral rotation, five of which arise from the pubis, the ischium, or both, one from the sacrum and one, the gluteus maximus (page 51) from the iliac crest, sacrum and coccyx. One, the piriformis, crosses the sacroiliac articulation.

Insertion: All insert into the trochanteric fossa, greater trochanter, linea quadrata, gluteal tuberosity, or iliotibial band.

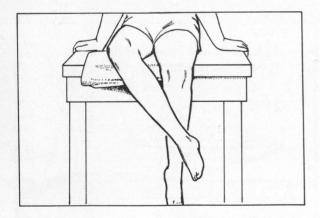

TEST FOR LATERAL ROTATORS OF THE HIP

In the sitting position, with legs over padded table edge and pelvis stabilized by grasping edge of table, rotate the thigh medially. The subject should approximate 45 degrees.

EVALUATION OF LIMITED MOTION

FLEXORS OF THE KNEE

Hamstrings

Biceps femoris (long head)
Origin: Ischial tuberosity.
Biceps femoris (short head)
Origin: Lateral lip of linea aspera, lateral supracondylar line of femur.
Insertion: Both muscles into head of fibula and lateral condyle of tibia.

Semitendinosus

Origin: Ischial tuberosity.
Insertion: Anteromedial surface of proximal end of tibia.

Semimembranosus

Origin: Ischial tuberosity.
Insertion: Posteromedial aspect of medial condyle of tibia.

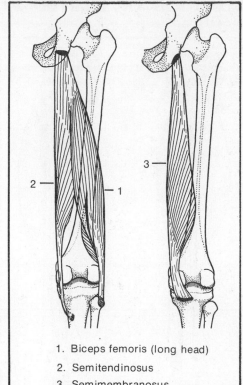

1. Biceps femoris (long head)
2. Semitendinosus
3. Semimembranosus

TEST FOR KNEE FLEXORS

In the supine position, with the arms straight and comfortably away from sides, flex one lower extremity as far as possible without bending the knee. The opposite extremity, which helps to keep the pelvis from tilting posteriorly, must stay in contact with the table. Seventy degrees of flexion is a reasonable amount.

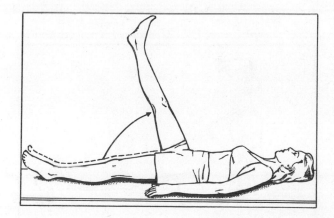

Alternate Test

Long-sitting position with the legs fully extended. The lower trunk is flexed forward as far as possible, avoiding flexion of the knees. The pelvis should approach a vertical position, about a 70 degree angle with the femur (not illustrated).

EVALUATION OF LIMITED MOTION

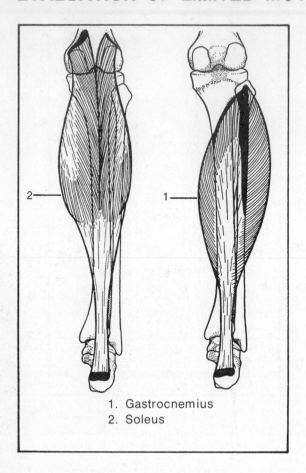

1. Gastrocnemius
2. Soleus

PLANTAR FLEXORS OF ANKLE

Gastrocnemius

Origin: Medial and lateral heads from medial and lateral condyles of femur.

Insertion: Tendo calcaneus, into posterior surface of calcaneus.

Soleus

Origin: Head and proximal third of fibular shaft, popliteal line, and middle third of tibia.

Insertion: Tendo calcaneus into posterior surface of calcaneus.

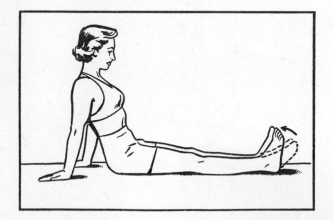

TEST FOR PLANTAR FLEXORS OF ANKLE

Gastrocnemius and Soleus

Long-sitting position, leaning backward to relax the tension in the posterior thigh muscles and fascia. With the knees straight, subject should be able to dorsiflex both ankles to a right angle.

Note: Examination of the metatarsal area of the feet may conveniently be combined with this test.

ANALYSIS OF BASIC ACTIVITIES

Name _____ Birth date _____

Date					Remarks with date
Sitting —balance					
—alignment					
Sitting to standing and return					
—Balance					
—Coordination					
—Use of arms					
—Foot placement					
Walking —Balance					
—Trunk position					
—Arm swing					
—Step length					
—Step rhythm					
—Foot placement					
Key — normal 1 good R right 2 fair L left 3 poor					Note: See section on Gait in *Muscle Testing* for detailed information

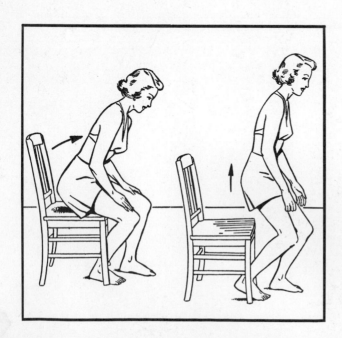

SITTING ALIGNMENT AND BALANCE

Use a chair that has sufficient width and breadth in the seat to provide even sitting support and that allows flexion of hips and knees to 90 degrees without pressure under the knees.

From the anterior view, note asymmetry demonstrated by an uneven level of head, shoulder, or pelvis. From the lateral view, note any forward shift of head or trunk. Record any difficulty in balance.

SITTING TO STANDING

Note first the base of support. A position with knees apart and one foot under chair with the heel off the floor and the other foot forward offers a wide base which helps maintain balance.

Record the use of the hands to aid weak knee and hip extensors or to assist in maintaining stability. Assistance will be required if the chair seat is low.

Note balance and coordination of motion.

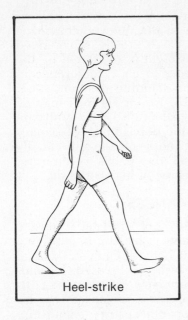

Heel-strike

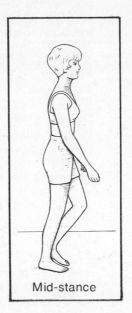

Mid-stance

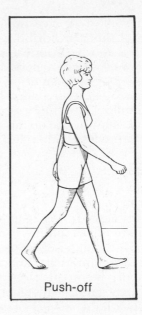

Push-off

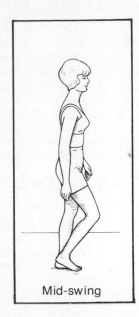

Mid-swing

WALKING*

First, observe the overall appearance. In the normal walking pattern the head and trunk are vertical, the arms swinging freely and in alternation with leg swing; step length and timing are even and the body oscillates vertically with each step.

At heel-strike, the foot is approximately at a right angle to the leg. The knee is extended but not locked in readiness for slight flexion as the body weight is shifted forward into the stance phase.

During stance, the trunk is maintained in the vertical position.

At push-off, the foot is strongly plantar flexed, with definite hyperextension of the metatarsophalangeal joints of the toes.

During the swing, the foot easily clears the floor with good alignment. The rhythm of movement remains unchanged.

*More detailed information concerning gait can be found in *Muscle Testing*, pages 153–163.

ADDITIONAL DATA FOR THE RECORD

CHEST EXPANSION

Expansion of the chest is measured to give an indication of thoracic flexibility. If this record is desired as a basis for estimating increase in mobility over a period of time, a simple procedure is to enter on the chart the difference in chest circumference between full expiration and full inspiration. This measurement is taken at the level of the xiphoid process with a flexible steel tape measure.

LEG LENGTH

If a difference in hip height is found, or for any reason asymmetry in leg length is suspected, measurements should be taken. The distance from the anterior superior spine of the ilium to the internal malleolus (ASSIM) is commonly recorded. Here the examiner should first stand at the foot of the table, grasp beneath the subject's heels, and pull downward on both extremities with an even traction to eliminate any asymmetry in pelvic position. After straightening the pelvic and leg alignment, the examiner may "match" the two inner malleoli to estimate any difference in leg length. The AAIM distance is then measured with a flexible steel tape. A good method is to fit one thumb, holding the tape, in the notch just below the anterior superior iliac spine and the other thumb in the depression just distal to the internal malleolus; the apex of these bony prominences may also be used. The exact procedure is a matter of individual preference.

Some persons consider a measurement of leg length taken in a nonweight-bearing position to have little practical value. Deviations such as foot pronation, knock knee, hyperextended knee, and so on sometimes appear unilaterally with weight bearing

and cause the leg to be "functionally" shorter. These deviations may be present to some degree in the nonweight-bearing position, but become greatly exaggerated when the body weight is supported by the extremity. In order to check difference in leg length in the standing position, small wood lifts of 1/16, 1/8, or 1/4 inch may be slipped under the foot of the extremity on the low side of the pelvis until it becomes level. The thickness of the lift finally required to level the pelvis is then recorded as the degree of leg shortenng.

MUSCLE WEAKNESS

The possibility of isolated muscle weakness must always be kept in mind in a general check of body alignment. Manual muscle strength tests can be used to evaluate muscle performance (see *Muscle Testing*). "Spotty" weakness, which may appear without any apparent cause, should be suspected, particularly in the presence of deviations such as head tilt, shift in trunk balance, scoliosis, pelvic asymmetry, unilateral leg malalignment, and uneven gait. Correction in these cases requires specific exercises for development of strength in the involved muscles.

MALALIGNMENT

So far in this chapter, most of the deviations from normal alignment that have been discussed might be said to fall within "physiologic" limits. While some degree of malalignment exists in these conditions and the body segments are not well balanced in relation to gravity, at the same time no deformity may yet be present that might be considered truly pathologic. It is difficult to draw a sharp line between the two, as this difference may be a matter of degree. The possibility is always present that so-called "physiologic" deviations not accompanied by pain may eventually deteriorate into painful and disabling conditions in which structural changes have taken place in the tissue.

OTHER DATA

Nutritional status, presence of neuromuscular tension, frequent or chronic fatigue, or disturbances of the patient's mental outlook that might conceivably influence his posture should be recorded. Height and weight may be included if this is not available elsewhere in the person's record.

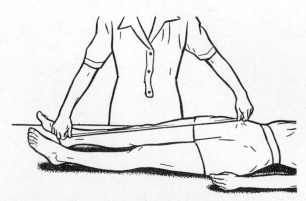

Figure 9. Leg length measurement.

II PLANNING THE EXERCISE PROGRAM

The exercise progressions presented are designed for the treatment of persons with those deviations in body alignment affecting function that have been detected by the evaluation procedures previously described. Deviations that are severe, of course, require concentrated attention. However, the potential for change of a slight or moderate degree of deviation to one resulting in disability should not be ignored when planning the exercise program. The "ideal" body alignment described in the plumb line tests used for posture evaluation is rarely reached. Much will depend on the kind, severity, and duration of impairment as well as on the age, body configuration, and environment of the individual.

Although patients are often referred to the exercise program for the relief of pain or the improvement of function in a limited segment of the body, the therapist has a responsibility to evaluate the total alignment and function of the patient in sufficient detail to provide knowledge of any possible contributory factors to the immediate problem. He is then in a position to develop an effective program for the patient.

OBJECTIVES

The general objective of the exercise program is to use kinesiological principles for the correction of any malalignment of the body that affects function or may lead to disability.

The specific objectives of the program are to:
1. Develop the kinesthetic sense of good alignment.
2. Relax unneeded musculature to permit smooth, coordinated, efficient motion.
3. Increase muscular strength as needed to attain and maintain good alignment and function.
4. Achieve flexibility within a normal range and the potential for change of the individual.

TOOLS

There are three tools available to the patient and his instructor for the accomplishment of the stated objectives:
1. Exercises for the development of kinesthetic sense, coordination, and strength.
2. Relaxation procedures for abnormal muscular tension.
3. Mobilization techniques for limited motion.

General mobilization exercises combine the above three elements. For example, while head and shoulder circling require muscle contraction, they also aid in relaxation of the muscles opposing each phase of the movement, and at the same time help to restore normal range of motion, which may be limited as the result of disease, injury, or poor habits of posture.

Special factors requiring consideration are the alleviation of pain and the tensions (from whatever cause) that require relaxation.

PAIN

The limiting factor in exercise is often pain. This is particularly so in the geriatric patient. The degree to which pain should be a contraindication to exercise is difficult to assess, as it depends upon the person's level of apprehension and tension as well as on the specific problem or problems for which the exercise program is undertaken. Muscle soreness due to disuse may be expected for a time; however, an increase in pain is a signal for a decrease in the difficulty of the exercises and, if persistent, a recheck with the referring physician.

The mechanisms that cause irritation resulting in pain and disability are graphically described by Cailliet (Fig. 10). The determination of the cause of pain and the means for its alleviation may be the first requirements for the exercise program. Here, techniques of conscious relaxation are particularly important.

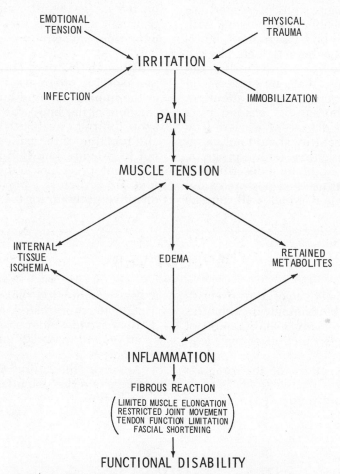

Figure 10. Mechanisms by which irritations result in functional disability. (From Cailliet, R.: Neck and Arm Pain. Philadelphia, F. A. Davis Co. 1964.)

RELAXATION

For some subjects it may be more difficult to acquire the ability to relax than to perform the exercises. Attention to the following aspects of the exercise program can assist the patient to relax.

First, relaxation after each exercise as well as between groups of exercises is essential, particularly if the subject has some degree of muscle tension in the region of the body concerned. The patient may be told to work as though each exercise were the last in the series and to pretend that he will be all through at the end of each exercise. This helps to eliminate the common tendency to maintain partial muscle contraction between exercises in anticipation of the next movement. The therapist must insist on controlled, deliberate action.

Second, if the patient appears to be overtense and has difficulty relaxing he may benefit from short rest periods before and during the exercise period. If this general tension is marked, specific training in a few procedures on the order of Jacobson's method to teach conscious relaxation may be indicated. For example, a child may be told to imagine he is melting like butter, or try to be a rag doll.

Third, the therapist should be alert to any evidence of marked emotional disturbance or economic pressures that may be contributing to the tensions of the patient and that may require assistance from other professional services. Often the therapist is in the best position of any person on the health team to observe these problems because of prolonged and relatively informal contact with the patient.

Fourth, the exercise activity should be well localized, using as few muscles as possible to perform the motion, and relaxing the remainder. This necessitates careful attention to adequate support and protection of the body segments required for the movement.

MOBILIZATION

TYPES OF PROCEDURES

When range of motion is limited, the type of procedure to be used in lengthening shortened muscles and their related connective tissue components is selected on the basis of effectiveness in the treatment of the disabling factors. The types commonly used are as follows:
1. Passive—application of external force without active movement.
2. Active assistive—contraction of the antagonist of the muscle to be elongated assisted by an external force applied manually by the therapist or with equipment.
3. Active—contraction of the antagonist of the muscle to be elongated.
4. Active resistive—contraction of the antagonist or agonist resisted manually or with equipment.

Passive mobilization is used primarily for those individuals who are unable to actively move the part or when active motion is contraindicated. All muscles involved are relaxed. The passive motions should be done slowly and carefully, as rapid movement activates the stretch reflex in the muscle being elongated and, if pain is elicited, a protective active contraction occurs. Both reactions are inhibiting forces that limit the range of motion.

Active assistive stretching is used for individuals who cannot actively complete the movement. They should be encouraged to try to assist throughout the range, as even a minimal contraction will effect some degree of relaxation in the shortened muscle (reciprocal innervation). Also, it leads to an increase in the strength of the antagonist, which is of primary importance in maintaining range of motion.

Active stretching may be done when the individual has sufficient strength in the antagonist to exert tension on the shortened muscle. Since no assistance or resistance is required, it can be carried out in the home as well as in the clinic to either maintain or gain range. Also, in contrast to the passive or active assistive types, active stretching is completely controlled by the individual; therefore, with proper instruction, too much force is not likely to be applied.

Active resistive stretching may be used when the individual has sufficient strength to resist an opposing force. It is helpful because, with careful adjustment of resistance, the stretch reflex can almost entirely be eliminated. It also has the advantage of being under the control of the individual, which minimizes the possibility of damage to tissues.

Resistance to the agonist, the shortened muscle, as well as to the antagonist may be used.

Tanagawa has reported on the result of experimental work with healthy young adults using the PNF "hold-relax" procedure. He found it to be superior to passive stretching in increasing the length of hamstring muscles. The technique was described as the application of maximal resistance to an isometric contraction of the shortened muscles at the point of limitation. The diagonal positions described by Knott and Voss were used. The author states that the results may be explained by autogenic inhibitions, as defined by Ruch and Patton, coupled with an active stretch on the connective tissues joining the muscles to their attachments.

It would appear that in the use of resistance to the agonist (the shortened muscle), attention should also be given to concurrent exercise to strengthen the antagonist in order to retain the increased length achieved. Inability of the antagonist of a shortened muscle to fully contract is usually the cause of shortening. The importance of a balance between agonists and antagonists in maintaining alignment and as a protection to joints has been emphasized by many authors.

It should be noted that the type of stretching may vary from one treatment period to another, and that combinations can be used within one session. The particular type must be fitted to the individual's ability and his reaction to the procedure as well as to the disability.

It seems obvious that gravity is a constant external force that can be used for assistance or resistance by a change in the position of the individual being treated.

EXTENSIBILITY OF CONNECTIVE TISSUE

Attention has been given to research on connective tissue. Kottke and his co-workers reported, on the basis of a clinical study, that moderate, sustained force used to increase range of motion produced better results than short-term, vigorous movement. He presented the concept that connective tissue placed under prolonged mild tension shows plastic elongation. This has been attributed to the separation of the attachments at the points of contact of collagen fibers in the connective tissue network. However, connective tissue has a very high tensile resistance to a suddenly applied force of short duration. For this reason, it can withstand high tensions exerted during strenuous muscular activity.

Warren and his collaborators report similar results from a laboratory study. Prolonged moderate stretching produced significantly greater residual length in collagenous tissue than did short-term, vigorous movements. Elevation of tissue temperature increased the efficacy of the procedure.

DURATION AND AMOUNT OF FORCE

It is apparent that in attempting to gain normal range of motion, we are concerned with complex physiological phenomena. Active stretching brings about relaxation in the shortened muscle through reciprocal innervation. Pain can trigger a protective active muscle contraction. Vigorous force applied rapidly activates both the stretch reflex in muscle and the guarding reaction of connective tissue. Also, it should be noted that extreme vigor can damage muscle fibers and other soft tissues, and the excessive use of outside force can bring about serious injury to joint surfaces and bony structures.

In carrying out the active stretching exercises presented in this text, the part should be slowly carried through as full a range of motion as is possible with a moderate muscle contraction, the position then held for a few seconds, followed by relaxation. On each repetition, a slight increase in range should be attempted. On the final effort, the contraction should be maintained for a longer period of time before relaxation.

THE EXERCISE PROGRAM

Starting with exercises for improving the specific area of impairment is the generally accepted approach to therapeutic exercise. The time available for the program necessitates this pattern. However, the "ideal" goal of total body balance and efficient function must be kept in mind by both subject and therapist. A few moments at the beginning or end of the exercise session spent on the development of an improved postural awareness of good position in standing, sitting, or moving positions can contribute to the more rapid translation of the exercise program into improved function of the total body.

Full recognition should be given to the fact that establishing an awareness of improved alignment and developing the ability and strength to use it effectively takes not days or weeks but months. Many exercise programs are undertaken for the alleviation of painful symptoms and are discontinued when this objective has been attained, with the result that recurrence of the symptoms is not infrequent. Factors that need to be considered in the exercise program follow.

PROGRESSION IN DIFFICULTY

Exercises for individual segments of the body should begin with those performed easily, requiring a minimum of strength and coordination. More strenuous and difficult exercises may be introduced as soon as indicated, until alignment of the whole body at once is possible through a combination of movements. Progression must be suited to the individual and should be instituted only as fast as the patient can learn to do more difficult activities in good form. If the exercise cannot be performed well, an easier exercise should be substituted for a time. Thus, the therapist must constantly adapt each fundamental exercise into easier or more difficult procedures as needed.

KINESIOLOGICAL FACTORS IN PROGRESSION

An understanding of the kinesiological factors of progression: gravitational forces, angle of application of forces, muscle length, and passive tension of two-joint muscles is basic to the understanding and planning of the exercise program.

GRAVITATIONAL FORCES

In planning a satisfactory exercise progression for the patient, not only must the anatomical position of the muscles and joint structures be considered but also the mechanics of motion must be understood and applied. For example, the center of gravity of the parts involved must be kept in mind. Many exercises involving trunk or leg raising can be made more or less difficult by varying the weight distribution. Trunk raising or "sit-ups" may be done first with the hands at the sides and later with the hands on the hips, then with the forearms folded across the abdomen, hands on opposite shoulders, clasped behind the neck, on top of the head and, finally, extended overhead. This upward shift of arm weight serves to move the center of gravity (of the entire portion raised) toward the head by stages, and thereby progressively to increase the difficulty of the exercise. If in performing trunk raising the patient is allowed to "roll up" by flexing his cervical and thoracic spine first, he will find it much easier than if he tries to keep his spine straight. Stabilization of the legs will be required if there is greater weight in the trunk and shoulders (Fig. 11).

Leg raising exercises may be done in the

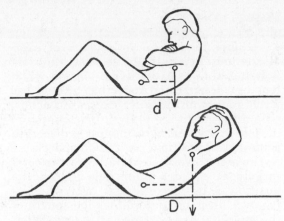

Figure 11. Trunk raising. Gravitational force increases as the distance between the axis of motion and the center of gravity of the portion of the body which is raised is increased. D > d.

supine position, first with the knees completely flexed, then partially flexed, and eventually fully extended for maximum resistance (Fig. 12). Likewise, in prone lying exercises for strengthening of the scapular adductor muscles, raising the arms with the elbows flexed will give less resistance than if the arms are nearly or completely straight.

ANGLE OF APPLICATION OF FORCE

Another consideration is the effectiveness of the angle of application of muscular and gravitational forces. A muscle pulling at or near a right angle to the long axis of the segment exerts its force more effectively than when its angle of pull is very small. Likewise, the force of gravity on a segment is maximal when the part is horizontal, and diminishes as it moves toward the vertical. Consequently, trunk flexion or leg flexion in the supine position is more difficult at the beginning of the movement and becomes easier as the motion progresses. Also, leg abduction is more difficult in the sidelying position than in standing.

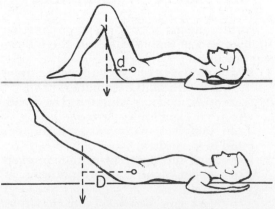

Figure 12. Leg raising.

41

MUSCLE LENGTH

An important factor in analysis of exercise is muscle length. In general, a muscle is better able to exert active tension when it is in a lengthened state than after it has undergone considerable shortening. Thus, when it is desirable to limit the action of a muscle in a given movement it is placed in a shortened position, or "put on a slack."

The active tension exerted by a two-joint muscle at a given joint depends on the position of the second joint over which it passes, since this determines the length of the muscle. For instance, the hamstrings are more effective as knee flexors when the hip is flexed and less effective when the hip is extended. Similarly, the gastrocnemius is a poor plantar flexor of the foot when the knee is flexed.

PASSIVE TENSION OF TWO-JOINT MUSCLES

The part played by passive tension of two-joint muscles in controlling the range of joint motion is another important kinesiologic factor in the analysis of exercise. The hip can be flexed to only 70 to 90 degrees if the knee is straight but considerably more if the knee is flexed, in which position the hamstrings are relaxed. The ankle flexes to slightly above a right angle with the knee straight but through an additional 20 to 30 degrees of motion if the gastrocnemius is relaxed by knee flexion. These considerations are particularly important in planning effective stretching procedures and also in analyzing necessary stabilization of the body segments in all types of exercise.

OTHER FACTORS IN PROGRESSION OF EXERCISES

Further means of controlling progression in the exercise regimen include the following practices:

1. Performing an exercise with one extremity, then with both extremities.
2. Increasing or decreasing the speed with which an exercise is performed. (A medium rate is usually easier than very rapid or very slow.)
3. Increasing the range of motion in exercises such as double knee circling.

4. Increasing the number of times an exercise is performed or the number of exercises in a series.
5. Decreasing the rest interval and lengthening the periods of activity.
6. Combining several exercises, thus saving time and increasing the difficulty of performance.
7. Changing the starting position of an exercise from recumbency (prone, supine, or side lying) to sitting, standing, or walking as soon as control of the body segments has been acquired.

For all persons undertaking corrective programs, exercises relating to their daily activities should be sought. For example, those driving long distances can do exercises requiring "gluteal pinch," scapular adduction, and correction of spinal alignment with considerable alleviation of tension and fatigue. Desk workers can do similar exercises plus head and shoulder movements. The ingenious therapist and patient can work out many supplementary activities to a prescribed exercise program which will relate to the individual's particular problems and environment.

PRECAUTIONS

The importance of physiological and mechanical protection of the patient while undertaking an exercise program cannot be overemphasized. Balance of segmental weights, protection against strain of one body segment while exercising another, and breath control are typical examples.

Very strenuous exercises should be used with great selectivity. For example, trunk raising from the supine position and double leg raising with knees extended are contraindicated for patients with back disabilities because of the strain on the low back from the contraction of the powerful hip flexors. Also, they are seldom used for older patients or for those with any form of debility who might become exhausted. Other exercises that accomplish the same purpose can be selected. Consideration of these factors is included in the presentation of the exercises.

In the home situation, it is not practical to suggest that elderly patients or those with back disabilities carry out exercises on the floor, because of the difficulty in getting up and down and the danger in falling. A bed with a firm mattress (bed board if needed) is satisfactory.

In the treatment center, a padded table or platform with more length and breadth than the standard treatment table is helpful. The added dimensions give a greater sense of security to the person who has a disturbance of balance. If the table is the height of a standard bed or a dining room chair seat, it is easier for the patient to go from a sitting position to lying or standing.

THE THERAPIST AS A TEACHER

Motivation is a primary factor in treatment and may be stimulated in many ways as in the following examples:
1. Assisting the patient to understand his own problems and the objective of each of his exercises. A progress check from time to time stimulates further effort.
2. Pointing out improvement rather than shortcomings as a more effective procedure. This tactic should be guided by the patient's personality and reaction to suggestions.
3. Having patients work in pairs or small groups for added stimulation. An element of play for younger patients and competition for older persons is helpful. Individual attention, however, should not be neglected through overemphasis on group activity.

The response of the subject to exercise therapy is also influenced to a large degree by the attitude and technique of the instructor. Clear, simple directions should be given. It will be learned quickly which directions have meaning for the patient and which do not. Preliminary explanations should not be so lengthy that the person loses the train of thought before starting the activity. It may be more satisfactory to give step-by-step directions as the exercise is being performed. The instructor should give the person his full attention. His own assurance and confidence will be reflected in the person's confidence and pleasure in working with him.

Finally, the instructor's own body alignment is important, both as a good example to patients and co-workers and from the very practical aspect of protecting himself against strain and injury.

POSITIONS FOR STARTING EXERCISES

When selecting a starting position for an exercise, the following points should be considered: the presence of pain or discomfort, the ability of the patient to assume the position, the use of a short lever arm versus a long lever arm, the need to stabilize one segment of the body to permit safe and efficient movement of another, and the use of gravity for assistance or resistance. Basic starting positions for therapeutic exercises are presented on the following pages.

Hooklying

This is a basic position for leg-raising exercises in which a short lever arm is desirable. In addition, the contraction of abdominal muscles can be emphasized with less hip flexor activity for both leg raising and trunk and neck flexion.

Knees are flexed to 90 degrees or more; soles of feet on table.

Arms may be placed in a position to exert counterpressure, or as a counterbalance, or to add to the length of the lever arm according to individual need.

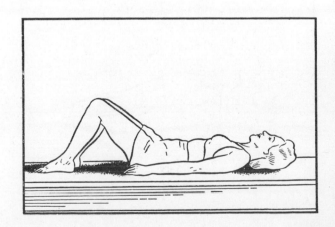

POSITIONS FOR STARTING EXERCISES

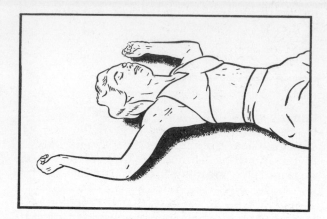

Hooklying, Arms Reverse T

This position maintains good shoulder alignment

Elbows are at a right angle, arms are abducted to 90 degrees and completely rotated laterally. Tension is placed on the pectoralis major muscles, which elevate the chest wall. Medial rotators of the shoulder are elongated and the scapulae adducted. Downward pressure on the elbows provides lateral stabilization for trunk and leg movements and the weight of the arms acts as a counterbalance for leg activities. Additional stability can be obtained by grasping the edge of the table or, when on a mat, the legs of a stool, chair, or table.

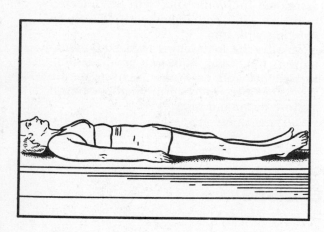

Backlying

Hips and knees are extended, the back is flat, and the neck is in axial extension. Arms are at sides, palms in contact with table. The arms may be abducted approximately 45 degrees, with elbows partially flexed to increase lateral stability by counterpressure during leg-raising exercises and rotation of the lower trunk.

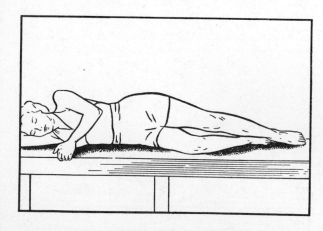

Sidelying

The lower leg is flexed approximately 45 degrees at hip and knee for balance, and the upper leg is extended. The arm beneath the trunk may be fitted into the space between the thorax and the ilium or placed under the head. The upper arm is used for balance and to prevent trunk rotation.

POSITIONS FOR STARTING EXERCISES

Facelying

The hips and knees are extended, the arms at the sides, abducted or rotated, or in reverse T position. The head lies to one side.

The head may be face down, resting on the forehead with chin tucked in when shoulder girdle exercises or extension of the thoracic and cervical spine is to be undertaken. A folded towel under the forehead may add to the comfort of the patient in this position.

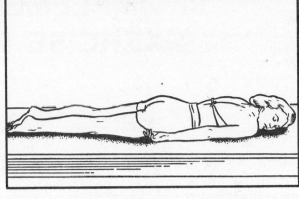

Long Sitting

The knees are extended and the ankles relaxed; the weight of the trunk is partially supported by the arms. Keep the spine in good alignment (knees slightly flexed if hamstrings are tight to avoid lumbar strain). Shoulders are adducted (not hunched).

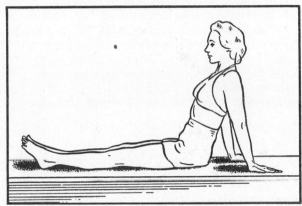

Hook Sitting

The knees are flexed, and the soles of the feet are flat on the plinth. The weight of the trunk is partially supported on the arms. The head and trunk are maintained in good alignment.

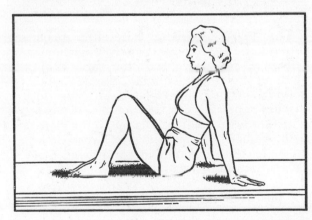

Cross Sitting (Tailor or Indian Sitting)

The hips are abducted and externally rotated; the feet are crossed and resting on lateral borders. The neck is in axial extension, the thoracic spine extended, and the arms relaxed at sides.

The lumbar spine is well fixed in this position, giving stability and balance to the trunk and providing firm support for shoulder, arm, head and trunk movements.

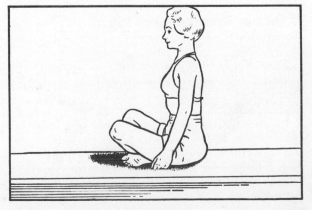

III IMPLEMENTING THE EXERCISE PROGRAM

Various types of exercises, in addition to the "active" type presented in this book, are used extensively by therapists. Passive, active assistive, and active resistive are the most common ones. In this book, the placement of the anatomic illustrations adjacent to the exercises makes it possible to determine the line of muscle contraction for assistance, resistance, and stabilization. The companion text, *Muscle Testing*, by the same authors covers range of motion, hand placement for resistance and stabilization, and additional positions for exercise. It is not practical to repeat them here.

Systems of exercise, such as proprioceptive neuromuscular facilitation (PNF) and progressive resistance exercises, are not reviewed or discussed, for they are available in their entirety elsewhere.

THE PELVIS AND SPINE

PELVIC SEGMENT

The pelvic segment has often been termed the key to good body alignment. However, the pelvis and the three divisions of the spine —lumbar, thoracic, and cervical— are too interrelated in action to discuss separately. For example, a patient with a forward head usually has an increase in the thoracic curve but may have either an increase in the lumbar curve, with the pelvis anteriorly rotated, or a rounding of the entire spine, with the pelvis in a neutral position or even posteriorly rotated.

PLANES OF REFERENCE FOR PELVIC ALIGNMENT

Two planes of reference for the "normal" pelvic alighment of use in checking the standing position have been described by Steindler.

In the lateral view in Figure 13, one plane, from the symphysis pubis upward to the anterior superior iliac spines, is vertical. The other, from the anterior iliac spines to the posterior inferior iliac spines, is horizontal.

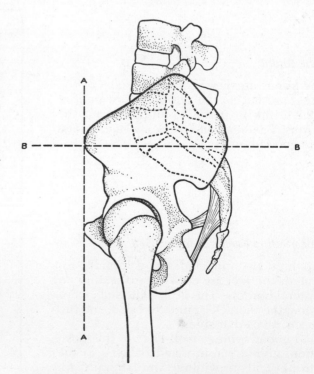

Figure 13. Lateral view of vertical and horizontal planes in normal pelvic alignment. *AA,* Anterior superior iliac spines to symphysis pubis; *BB,* anterior superior iliac spines to posterior inferior iliac spines.

ANTEROPOSTERIOR ROTARY STRESSES ON PELVIC AREA

As discussed earlier, the line of gravity of the suprafemoral part of the body usually falls slightly behind the axes of the hip joints. The spine rests on the posterior part of the pelvic ring and consequently exerts a rotary stress on the pelvic segment, which tends to push it down posteriorly. In spite of this, a common deviation is forward, or anterior, tilting of the pelvis, particularly if some degree of hyperextension of the knees is present. As the femur moves backward, tight hip flexor muscles and the anterior ligaments of the hip joint tend to pull the pelvis down anteriorly.

The base of the sacrum, upon which the spine is supported, is not horizontal but slants in an anterior direction. Thus, there is a shearing force exerted between the lumbar spine and the base of the sacrum. The distal lumbar vertebrae are prevented from sliding forward by the ligaments of the area, the fibrocartilaginous interverte-bral discs and the osseous vertebral arches (Fig. 14).

The sacrum itself is subjected to antero-posterior rotatory stresses, with a potential frontal axis passing through the auricular areas of the ilia. The thrust of the vertebral column tends to force the proximal end of the sacrum forward and downward: this displacement is resisted by the anterior and posterior sacroiliac ligaments. The corresponding upward and backward movement of the distal ends of the sacrum and coccyx is prevented by the very strong sacrospinous and sacrotuberous ligaments (Fig. 14).

The more the position of the sacrum approximates the horizontal plane the more the supraincumbent vertebral column is in a position to exert pressure, resulting in forward rotation of the sacrum. Hence, anterior sacral displacement is favored by anterior rotation of the pelvis or, conversely, each of these difficulties is less likely to occur with the pelvis tilted posteriorly. This is a most important concept in standing alignment (Fig. 15).

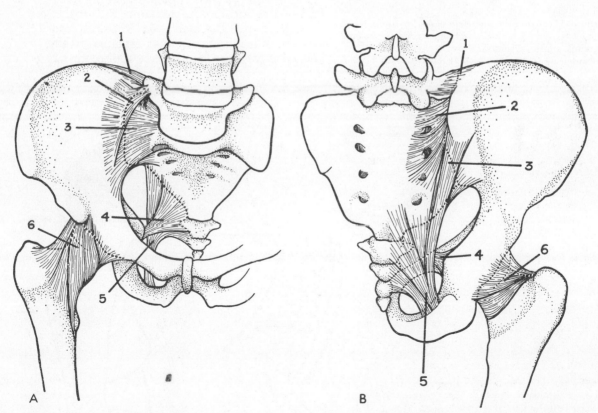

Figure 14. Ligaments of importance in the postural mechanics of the lumbosacral, sacroiliac and hip joints. A, Anterior view; *1*, iliolumbar; *2*, lumbosacral; *3*, anterior sacroiliac; *4*, sacrospinous; *5*, sacrotuberous; *6*, iliofemoral. B, Posterior view; *1*, iliolumbar; *2*, short posterior sacroiliac; *3*, long posterior sacroiliac; *4*, sacrospinous; *5*, sacrotuberous; *6*, ischiocapsular.

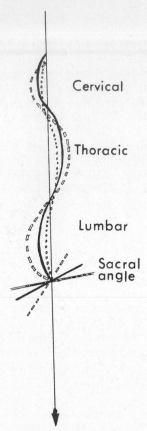

Cervical

Thoracic

Lumbar

Sacral
angle

Figure 15. Lateral view (*left,* anterior; *right,* posterior). Change of superincumbent curves influenced by sacral angle. (From Cailliet, R.: Low Back Pain Syndrome. Philadelphia, F. A. Davis Co., 1968.)

As the vertical line of the body falls anterior to the thoracic spine, gravitational force constantly tends to increase the normal posteriorly convex curve. This increase in curvature is opposed by the resistance to compression of the vertebral discs and by tension of the erector spinae muscles and posterior spinal ligaments.

Owing to the overlapping of the long, downward slanting, spinous processes of the thoracic vertebrae, the thoracic spine normally has no appreciable degree of hyperextension. The erector spinae, therefore, act not only as prime movers in spinal extension but also as fixators for movements such as raising the head and arms in prone-position exercises.

The positions of the thoracic and cervical spines are interrelated. If round back is present, the individual is very likely to have a forward head. As the thoracic curve is straightened, the head may be moved upward and backward into a corrected position, a movement which will be called here "axial extension" in order to avoid confusion with the correct meaning of the terms extension and hyperextension (Fig. 16).

Only in the thoracic area do the erector spinae muscles act alone as erectors. In the cervical region, their contraction brings

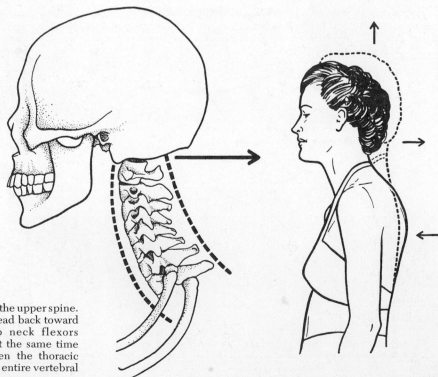

Figure 16. Axial extension of the upper spine. The neck extensors move the head back toward the midline while the deep neck flexors straighten the cervical spine. At the same time the thoracic extensors straighten the thoracic spine so that the alignment of the entire vertebral column is improved.

about neck hyperextension, with an upward tilting of the chin: in the low back these muscles shorten with hyperextension or lordosis. Straightening of the lumbar spine is accomplished by leveling of the pelvis through upward abdominal muscle pull anteriorly and downward hip extensor muscle pull posteriorly. Axial extension of the cervical spine involves a different mechanism.

CERVICAL SPINE

Certain head extensor muscles arising from the upper thoracic and lower cervical vertebrae exert an oblique pull on the head and neck in a downward and backward direction. If this line of pull falls behind the atlantooccipital joint, a rotary movement will result which tilts the head back and elevates the face, hyperextending the neck. If, however, this posterior head rotation is prevented by the neck flexors, the oblique pull may be seen to have a posterior translatory component when the head is forward, serving to pull the head back nearer to the vertical gravity line and into better alignment. (Neck flexors in this case include the rectus capitis anticus and the muscles pulling the chin toward the hyoid bone and the hyoid toward the thorax.) In addition, the longus colli and longus capitis muscles exert a direct bowstring action on the front of the cervical column, aiding in axial extension of the neck. Axial extension really consists of neck flexion or straightening of the anterior convexity of the cervical curve. This is performed best in combination with straightening the posterior convexity of the thoracic curve (Fig. 16).

EXERCISE PROGRESSION FOR ALIGNMENT OF PELVIC SEGMENT, SPINE AND SHOULDER GIRDLE

The most common deviations in the alignment of the trunk are an anterior rotation of the pelvis, an increase in the spinal curves, and a forward shift of the pelvic girdle. Correction involves flattening of the lumbar curve, axial extension of the neck, and flattening of the thoracic curve together with control of the shoulder girdle.

Exercise progressions for the alignment of the pelvic and spinal segments are presented in the following pages, coordinated with pertinent anatomical information. General precautions are summarized for each area. Specific precautions pertaining to an exercise are included in the description.

MUSCLES TO BE STRENGTHENED

TRUNK FLEXORS

Rectus Abdominis

Origin: Crest of pubis and adjacent ligaments.

Insertion: Cartilages of fifth, sixth and seventh ribs.

This muscle exerts a direct line of pull to correct anterior rotation (forward tilting) of the pelvis, with accompanying lordosis and strain on the low back structures. This muscle also supports and prevents protrusion of the anterior abdominal wall.

Obliquus Externus Abdominis

Origin: Lower eight ribs.

Insertion: Anterior half of iliac crest, pubic tubercle and pectineal line, and aponeurosis of opposite muscle forming linea alba, which extends from symphysis pubis to xiphoid process.

Obliquus Internus Abdominis

Origin: Lateral portion of inguinal ligament, anterior two thirds of iliac crest, and thoracolumbar fascia.

Insertion: Crest of pubis, linea alba, and cartilages of lower three or four ribs.

The oblique muscles act as rotators of the trunk, the pull of the external oblique on one side being continued through that of the internal oblique on the other. In this way the thorax is rotated in relation to the pelvis or the pelvis in relation to the thorax, depending on the fixation of the parts. The lateral portions of these muscles act in lateral trunk flexion as well as in forward flexion and help to prevent anterior pelvic tilt. The obliques are also powerful constrictors of the thoracic and abdominal cavities.

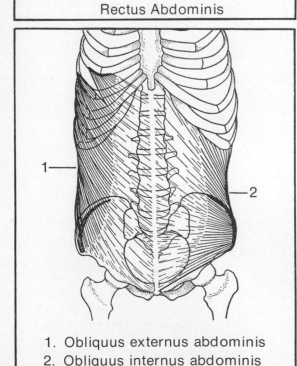

Rectus Abdominis

1. Obliquus externus abdominis
2. Obliquus internus abdominis

ALIGNMENT OF PELVIC SEGMENT AND LUMBAR SPINE

MUSCLES TO BE STRENGTHENED

HIP EXTENSORS

Gluteus Maximus

Origin: Posterior iliac crest, posterior sacrum and coccyx, sacrotuberous ligament.

Insertion: Gluteal ridge, between greater trochanter and linea aspera, and iliotibial band over greater trochanter.

This muscle, although primarily a hip extensor, in the weight bearing position (acting from its insertion) assists with the correction of anterior rotation of the pelvis.

Hamstrings

Semitendinosus
Origin: Ischial tuberosity.
Insertion: Anteromedial surface of proximal end of tibia.

Semimembranosus
Origin: Ischial tuberosity.
Insertion: Posteromedial aspect of medial tibial condyle.

Biceps femoris (Long head)
Origin: Ischial tuberosity.
Insertion: Lateral side head of fibula and lateral condyle of tibia.

The downward pull of the hamstring muscles is in a direct line to rotate the pelvis posteriorly. The rectus abdominis muscles anteriorly, together with the hamstring muscles posteriorly, form a force couple that serves to correct anterior pelvic tilt.

EXERCISE PRECAUTIONS

Trunk or leg flexion exercises in the supine position strongly activate the iliopsoas muscle (page 60), which pulls on the lumbar spine and lumbosacral junction. These areas are often the site of strain and injury. These flexion exercises should be done with caution and only after control of the area is developed through exercises using a shorter leverage arm (such as with the knees flexed or partial flexion of the trunk with the pelvis stabilized).

Likewise, asymmetrical exercises should

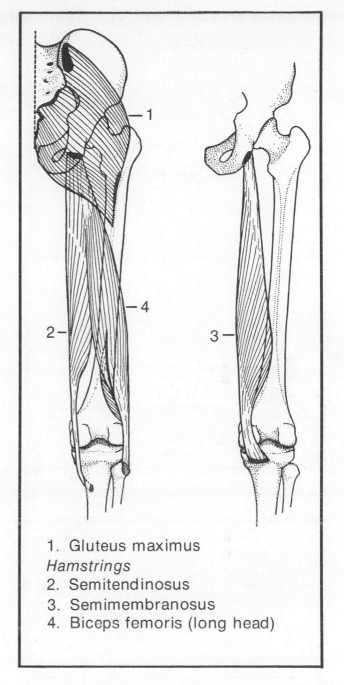

1. Gluteus maximus
Hamstrings
2. Semitendinosus
3. Semimembranosus
4. Biceps femoris (long head)

be avoided until pain has subsided and fairly vigorous exercises can be done with comfort and in good form.

When these exercises require considerable muscular effort there is a tendency to hold the breath (Valsalva effect), thus increasing intra-abdominal and intrathoracic pressure, with danger of abdominal or diaphragmatic hernia. The subject should exhale slowly, whistle, or count aloud during the exercise to make sure that the breath is not held.

ALIGNMENT OF PELVIC SEGMENT AND LUMBAR SPINE

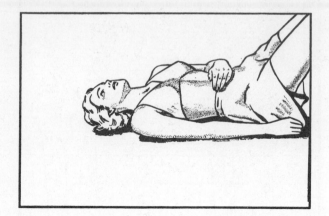

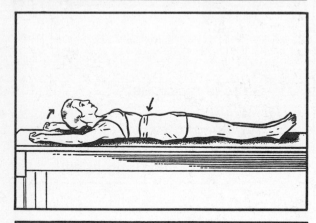

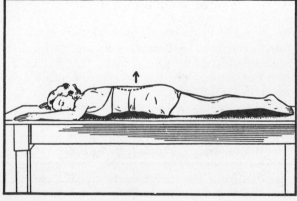

1. *Hooklying*
a. Hand on abdomen for palpation.
Contract abdominal muscles without attempting movement of pelvis or rib cage (muscle setting). Hold, then relax slowly.
b. Arms at sides.
Contract gluteal muscles (pinching) without attempting joint movement. Hold, then relax slowly.

2. *Hooklying*
a. Arms at sides.
Contract gluteal and abdominal muscles, rotating pelvis posteriorly and flattening lumbar spine (pelvic tilt). Hold, then relax slowly.
b. Progress through changes of arm position:
   1) abduct to 45, then to 90 degrees,
   2) use reverse T position (illustrated),
   3) abduct arms fully and extend elbows.
(If there is a tendency to hold breath, isolate pelvic motion from breathing cycle by holding rotation and breathing several times.)

3. *Hooklying*
a. Arms at sides.
Rotate pelvis posteriorly (pelvic tilt) and flex neck.
b. Progress to supine position.
c. Progress through changes in arm position (illustrated with reverse T).
(Head flexion may be added by pulling chin in as neck is flexed.)

4. *Prone lying*
a. Arms at sides.
Contract gluteal muscles. Hold, relax slowly and completely.
b. Contract abdominals strongly and relax.
c. Combine a and b, posteriorly rotating pelvis (pelvic tilt).
d. Progress through changes of arm position (illustrated with reverse T).
(Avoid tendency toward contraction of hip flexors.)

ALIGNMENT OF PELVIC SEGMENT AND LUMBAR SPINE

BASIC EXERCISES FOR CONTROL OF POSTERIOR PELVIC ROTATION

5. *Hooklying*

a. Arms at sides, slightly abducted.

Posteriorly rotate pelvis, flex one hip through range of motion and continue rotation until knee contacts chest. Hold pelvic tilt and return leg slowly to position.

b. Flex legs, bringing knees to chest. Hold pelvic tilt and return legs slowly to position.

c. Progress through changes in arm position (illustrated with reverse T).

(Counting out loud during all strenuous abdominal exercises prevents holding breath and increasing intra-abdominal pressure, Valsalva effect.)

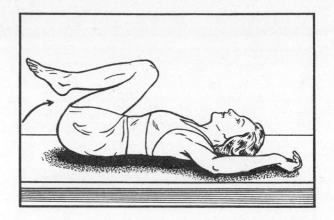

6. *Hooklying*

a. Arms at sides, slightly abducted.

Posteriorly rotate pelvis, hold, and slide one heel along table until hip and knee are extended. Return slowly to position.

b. Posteriorly rotate pelvis and slide both heels along table until legs are extended or until lumbar spine begins to arch.

c. Progress through changes in arm position (illustrated with reverse T).

(Further stabilization in the reverse T position is obtained by grasping the edge of the table or, if on mat, by grasping the legs of a chair or stool.)

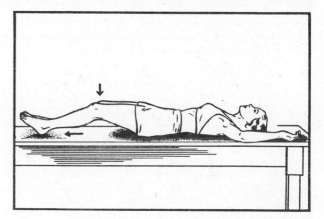

7. *Supine*, hips flexed to 90 degrees, knees completely flexed, arms abducted to 45 degrees or grasping table over head (latter illustrated).

a. Posteriorly rotate pelvis, hold, and make a small circle with knees. Alternate circle direction.

b. Progress to larger circles if strength permits and control can be maintained.

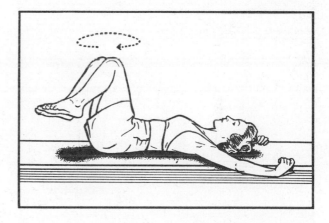

8. *Hooklying,* arms abducted to 45 degrees or grasping table over head (latter illustrated).

Flex hips bringing knees to chest (one), extend legs upward (two), flex again (three) and return to hooklying position (four).

The lumbar spine should remain in contact with table.

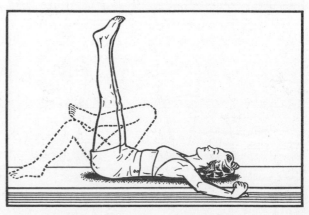

ALIGNMENT OF PELVIC SEGMENT AND LUMBAR SPINE

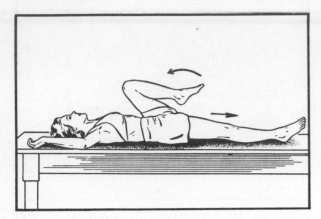

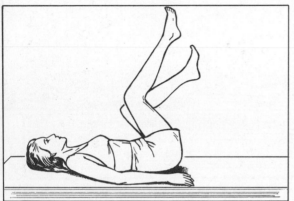

BASIC EXERCISES FOR CONTROL OF POSTERIOR PELVIC ROTATION

9. *Hooklying*
a. Arms at sides, slightly abducted.
Posteriorly rotate pelvis, flex one hip and knee and at the same time extend opposite leg until it rests on table. Return both extremities to position and alternate.
b. Progress through changes in arm position (illustrated with reverse T).

10. *Hooklying*
a. Arms abducted to 45 degrees or grasping table over head.
Flex hips, bringing both knees to chest. Partially extend one leg and then the other in a reciprocal leg circling or "bicycle" motion. Lower knees singly back to position.
b. Progress to larger circles if strength and control permit.

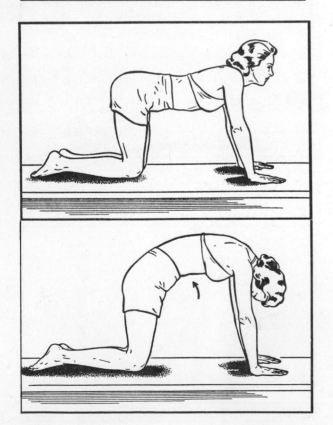

11. *Semi-prone*. Neck extended; shoulders, hips and knees flexed to 90 degrees; elbows extended; and weight on hands and knees.
Drop head and relax abdominal muscles, allowing lumbar spine to hyperextend.
Posteriorly rotate pelvis and flex trunk and neck through greatest possible range.
(If knees are sensitive, a small pad or pillow may be used.)

ALIGNMENT OF PELVIC SEGMENT AND LUMBAR SPINE

BASIC EXERCISES FOR CONTROL OF POSTERIOR PELVIC ROTATION

12. *Pronelying,* arms abducted with elbows extended.
a. Posteriorly rotate pelvis, hold, and raise each arm alternately from table. Return slowly to position.
b. Rotate pelvis, hold, and raise both arms from table. Hold for a specified count.

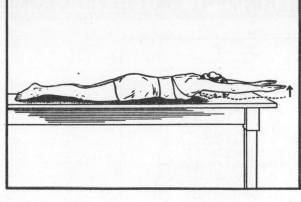

13. *Hooklying*
a. Arms at sides.
Posteriorly rotate pelvis, reach hands toward knees, and flex neck and trunk until lower borders of scapulae are off table. Lumbar spine should remain in contact with table.
b. Progress to arms crossed on chest (illustrated) and then with hands behind neck.

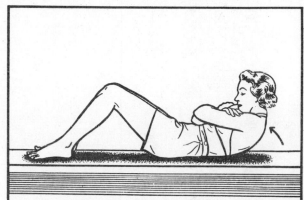

14. *Hooklying*
a. Arms at sides.
Posteriorly rotate pelvis, flex neck then trunk, continue with hip flexion, "rolling up" to a sitting position. Return to starting position, attempting to place each thoracic and cervical vertebra in sequence in contact with table.
b. Progress to arms crossed on chest (illustrated) and then with hands behind neck.

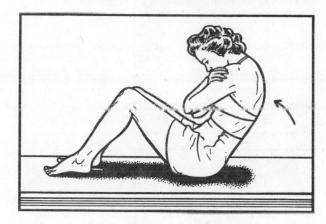

15. *Standing.*
a. Arms at sides, heels 4 to 6 inches from wall, trunk away from wall.
Lean backward, flex head (chin in) and attempt to flatten neck and spine against wall. Flex knees and slide trunk down the wall a few inches. Flatten the lumbar spine still more and return sliding up wall until knees are straight.
Next, lean forward from ankles and walk across room, maintaining position.
b. Repeat with hands behind neck and elbows touching wall (illustrated).
c. Place sand bag on top of head, arms relaxed at sides, and flatten spine against the wall. Lean forward, pushing up against weight, and walk across room.

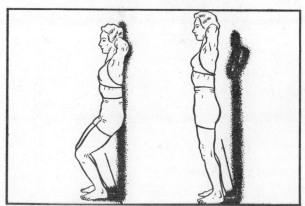

ALIGNMENT OF PELVIC SEGMENT AND LUMBAR SPINE

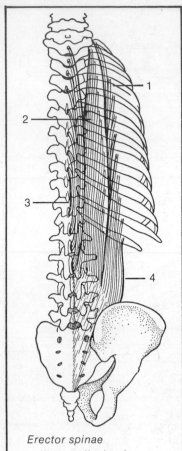

Erector spinae
1. Iliocostalis dorsi
2. Longissimus dorsi
3. Spinalis dorsi
4. Iliocostalis lumborum

LUMBAR EXTENSORS

Erector Spinae

Origin: Common tendon from posterior iliac crest, spinous processes of lower thoracic and lumbar vertebrae, and posterior aspect of the sacrum. The muscle group forms three vertical columns: The *iliocostalis, longissimus* and *spinalis.*

Insertion: Spinous and transverse processes of the cervical and thoracic vertebrae and adjacent area of ribs, mastoid process, and nuchal lines of the occipital bone. (Cervical and capitate portions are not illustrated.)

Because of the normal anteroposterior curves of the spine these muscles are truly erector spinae only in the thoracic area. In the lumbar area they increase the posterior concavity of the spine and oppose straightening of the column.

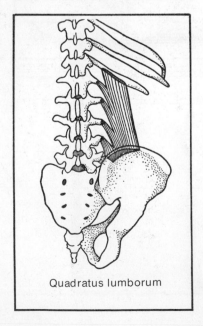

Quadratus lumborum

Quadratus Lumborum

Origin: Iliolumbar ligament and adjacent iliac crest.

Insertion: Medial one half of inferior border of last rib; transverse processes of first four lumbar vertebrae.

In the prone position, these muscles hyperextend and laterally flex the lumbar spine and, if shortened, limit correction of lordosis and scoliosis in this region.

ALIGNMENT OF PELVIC SEGMENT AND LUMBAR SPINE

SYMMETRICAL EXERCISES FOR STRETCHING SHORT LUMBAR EXTENSORS AND STRENGTHENING ABDOMINAL MUSCLES

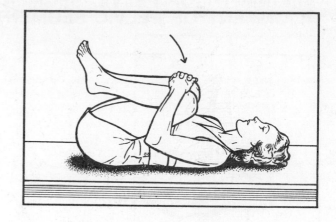

1. Supine, hips and knees flexed.
Posteriorly rotate pelvis, bringing knees toward chest.
Clasp hands around knees and pull tight to chest, keeping thoracic and cervical spine flat against table. Hold, then release handclasp slowly, attempting to maintain contraction of abdominal muscles.
Relax, repeat several times, then return to starting position.

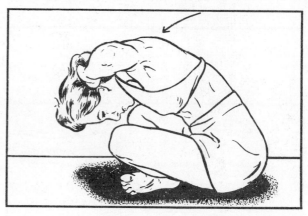

2. Cross sitting, hands behind neck.
Flex the hips, then the trunk with a contraction of the abdominal muscles. Hold, then repeat.
(If there is excessive flexion of the thoracic spine, keep neck straight with hands clasped behind back).

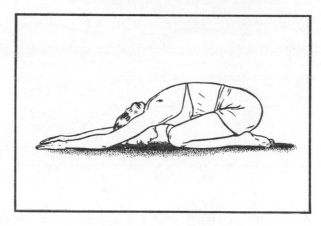

3. Crouch position, forehead resting on table and arms extended over head.
Lower chest toward knees. Push arms forward and contract abdominal muscles, forcing chest firmly against knees. Hold, then relax and repeat.

4. Sitting on chair, legs abducted (not illustrated).
Drop head and shoulders forward, flex hips, then contract abdominal muscles to flex trunk until shoulders are between knees. Hold, then repeat.

ALIGNMENT OF PELVIC SEGMENT AND LUMBAR SPINE

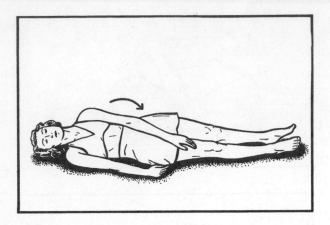

ASYMMETRICAL EXERCISES FOR STRETCHING SHORT LUMBAR EXTENSORS AND STRENGTHENING ABDOMINAL MUSCLES

1. Supine, arms at sides, pelvis posteriorly rotated.

Reach one hand toward opposite knee, keeping pelvis in contact with table Return slowly to starting position. Repeat to other side.

(Rotation of the trunk to one side with the pelvis fixed or rotation of the pelvis with the trunk flexed elongates the lumbar extensors of the opposite side.)

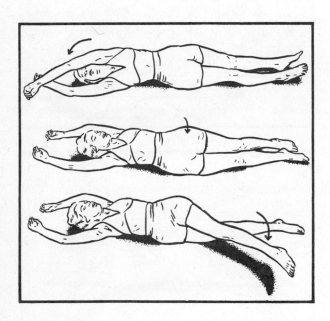

2. Supine or prone-lying, pelvis posteriorly rotated, arms extended over head.

(Exercise should be done on mat or floor.)

a. Lead with the arm and shoulder. Let the thorax rotate as far as possible before the pelvis and lower extremity follow.

b. Initiate the roll with the pelvic segment, letting the arm and leg follow.

c. Lead with the leg, the shoulder remaining in contact with the floor as long as possible. The leg is allowed to rotate inward to emphasize the rolling movement.

d. Progress to a series of rolls in each direction, if space permits, with a maximum range of motion.

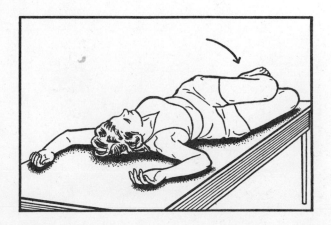

3. Hooklying, pelvis posteriorly rotated.

a. Arms abducted to 45 degrees.

Raise both knees until thighs are vertical. Lower knees toward the table on one side, maintaining shoulders in contact with table. Return knees slowly to vertical position. Repeat to other side.

b. Progress to reverse T position of arms (illustrated).

ALIGNMENT OF PELVIC SEGMENT AND LUMBAR SPINE

ASYMMETRICAL EXERCISES FOR STRETCHING SHORT LUMBAR EXTENSORS AND STRENGTHENING ABDOMINAL MUSCLES

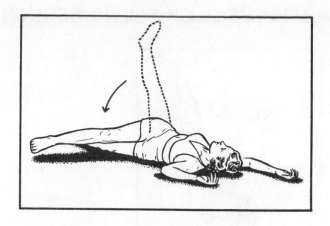

4. Supine, pelvis posteriorly rotated.
a. Arms abducted to 45 degrees.
Flex one hip until leg is near vertical, keeping shoulders flat to table. Touch foot to floor on opposite side of body at knee level. Return slowly to vertical position. Repeat, then change to opposite leg.
b. Progress to touching toe to floor near hip level. Keep shoulders as flat as possible.
c. Progress to reverse T position for arms (illustrated).

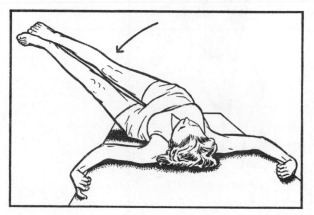

5. *Hooklying,* arms abducted to 45 degrees or grasping table over head, pelvis posteriorly rotated.
Flex hips until thighs are near vertical. Extend knees and lower legs toward floor on one side as far as possible while keeping shoulders flat on table.
Return slowly to vertical position, repeat, then change to opposite side.

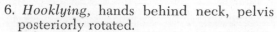

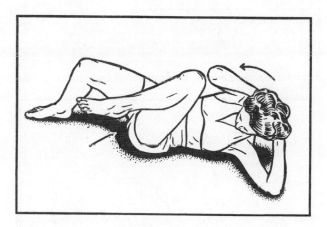

6. *Hooklying,* hands behind neck, pelvis posteriorly rotated.
a. Flex one hip and knee, flex trunk slightly, and rotate to touch opposite elbow to flexed knee.
Return slowly to position. Repeat, then change to opposite side.
b. Progress by sliding elbow along lateral side of flexed knee for more rotation. Do not allow elbow touching table to press downward.

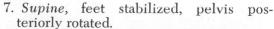

7. *Supine,* feet stabilized, pelvis posteriorly rotated.
a. Flex head and neck, reach one arm toward opposite knee and flex trunk with as much rotation as possible. Then flex hips, rolling up to a sitting position.
Return to supine, touching lumbar, thoracic, and cervical spines in succession (rolling up).
b. Progress to arms crossed on chest (illustrated), then hands behind neck.

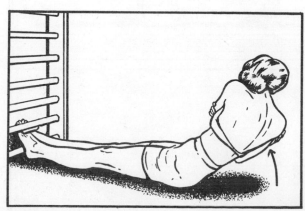

ALIGNMENT OF PELVIC SEGMENT AND LUMBAR SPINE

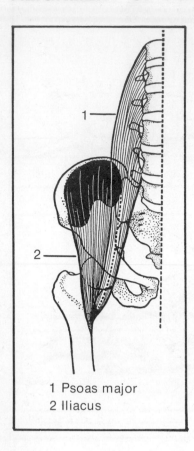

1 Psoas major
2 Iliacus

MUSCLES THAT MAY NEED STRETCHING

HIP FLEXORS

Psoas Major

Origin: Sides of bodies of last thoracic and all lumbar vertebrae, intervertebral fibrocartilages, and transverse processes of all lumbar vertebrae.

Insertion: Lesser trochanter of femur.

Iliacus

Origin: Upper two thirds of iliac fossa, inner lip of iliac crest, and base of sacrum.

Insertion: Body of femur below lesser trochanter and lateral side of tendon of psoas major.

The psoas major attaches to the lumbar spine, and thus is directly concerned in lordosis. Both trunk and leg flexion exercises in the supine position strongly activate the iliopsoas muscles, which pull on the lumbar spine and pelvis. The lumbosacral junction is so often the site of strain and injury that care must be taken to obtain adequate fixation of the lumbar spine and pelvis during stretches of this muscle.

EXERCISES FOR STRETCHING SHORT HIP FLEXORS.

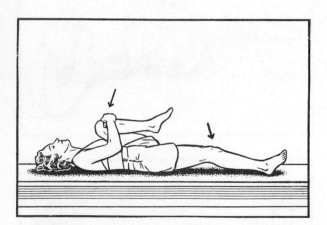

1. *Hooklying*

Flex one hip and knee and hold firmly against chest with hand clasp. Extend opposite leg, and attempt to flatten the back of the knee against table to lengthen hip flexors.

Keep thoracic spine extended.

ALIGNMENT OF PELVIC SEGMENT AND LUMBAR SPINE

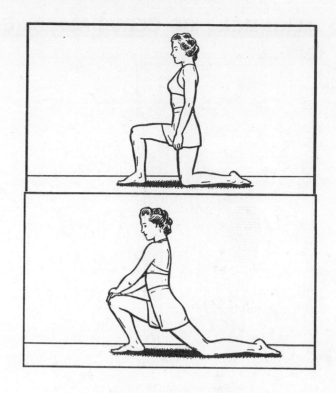

EXERCISES FOR STRETCHING SHORT HIP FLEXORS

2. *Kneeling*, hip and knee of one leg to right angle.

Lean trunk forward, increasing flexion of hip and knee to lengthen hip flexors of opposite leg.

Repeat, then change to other leg.

Spine is maintained in extension.

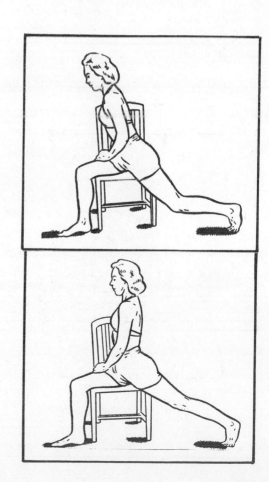

3. *Sitting*, edge of chair, supporting one thigh with hip and knee flexed to right angles. Opposite hip is extended as far as possible with knee partially flexed.

Extend knee, attempting to lengthen hip flexors on that side.

Repeat, then change sides.

Trunk is maintained in a vertical position.

ALIGNMENT OF CERVICAL SPINE

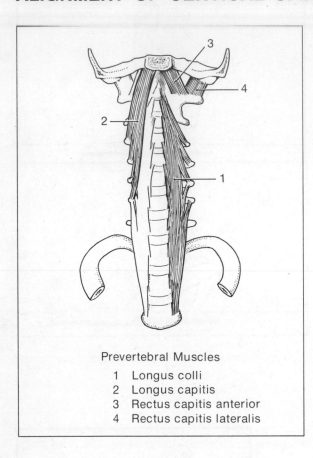

Prevertebral Muscles

1 Longus colli
2 Longus capitis
3 Rectus capitis anterior
4 Rectus capitis lateralis

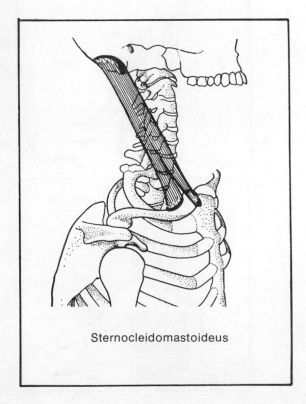

Sternocleidomastoideus

PREVERTEBRAL MUSCLES
(NECK FLEXORS)

Longus Colli and Capitis

Origin: Transverse processes of third to sixth cervical and first three thoracic vertebrae.

Insertion: Inferior surface basilar part of occipital bone, tubercle on anterior arch of atlas, transverse processes of fifth and sixth cervical, and anterior surface bodies of second to fourth cervical vertebrae.

Rectus Capitis Anterior

Origin: Anterior surface of lateral mass of atlas and transverse process.

Insertion: Inferior surface of basilar part of occipital bone.

Rectus Capitis Lateralis

Origin: Superior surface of transverse process of atlas.

Insertion: Inferior surface of jugular process of occipital bone.

The longus colli and capitis and the rectus capitis anterior and lateralis are direct antagonists of the muscles at back of the neck, serving to restore the head to a natural position after it has been drawn backward. They also flex the head. The rectus capitis lateralis, acting singly, bends the head laterally.

NECK FLEXOR

Sternocleidomastoideus

Origin: Upper anterior manubrium sterni; superior and anterior medial third of clavicle.

Insertion: Lateral surface of mastoid process and superior nuchal line of occipital bone.

If the prevertebral muscles are weak, the contraction of these muscles will increase rather than decrease the convexity of the cervical spine. The head can be raised from the supine position but will be rotated posteriorly, chin up ("turtle neck").

ALIGNMENT OF CERVICAL SPINE

MUSCLES TO BE STRENGTHENED

NECK EXTENSORS

Trapezius (Upper Fibers)

Origin: External occipital protuberance, medial third of superior nuchal line of the occiput, and the ligamentum nuchae.

Insertion: Posterior border of lateral third of clavicle.

By reverse action the upper trapezius extends the head.

Semispinalis Capitis

Origin: Transverse processes of the seventh cervical and first six or seven thoracic vertebrae.

Insertion: Nuchal line of the occipital bone.

Splenius Capitis

Origin: Caudal half of ligamentum nuchae, spinous processes of seventh cervical and first three or four thoracic vertebrae.

Insertion: Occipital bone just caudal to lateral third superior nuchal line and mastoid process of temporal bone.

Splenius Cervicis

Origin: Spinous processes of third to sixth thoracic vertebrae.

Insertion: Transverse processes of upper two or three cervical vertebrae.

Erector Spinae

Cervical and capitate sections not illustrated.

The cervical and capitate divisions of the erector spinae, together with the splenius capitis and cervicis and the semispinalis capitis, assist in axial exten-

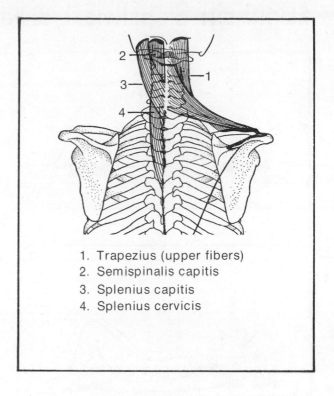

1. Trapezius (upper fibers)
2. Semispinalis capitis
3. Splenius capitis
4. Splenius cervicis

sion of the head by bringing the head back toward the midline of the body. Their hyperextension action must be counterbalanced by the prevertebral muscles (page 62).

(See discussion of axial extension, pages 48, 49 and 50.)

PRECAUTION

Careful localization of motion is necessary in exercises to correct a forward head. The movement should take place in the spine only above the apex of the posterior thoracic convexity. If too large an area is involved, lumbar extension may result rather than specific correction of the neck and head position.

ALIGNMENT OF CERVICAL SPINE

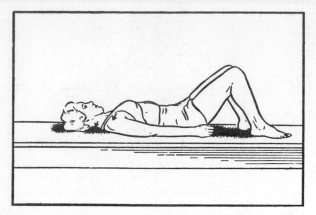

BASIC EXERCISES

1. *Hooklying,* arms at sides.
Stretch the back of the head toward the end of the table, keeping the chin in and flattening the cervical spine in axial extension. Keep the shoulders in contact with the table.
(For axial extension, see pages 48, 49, 50 and 63.)

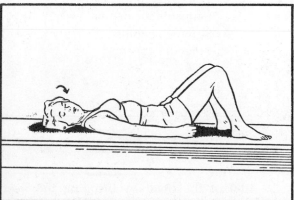

2. *Hooklying,* arms at sides.
Rotate the head toward one shoulder as far as possible, maintaining axial extension of the cervical spine.
Return to the starting position; repeat to other side.

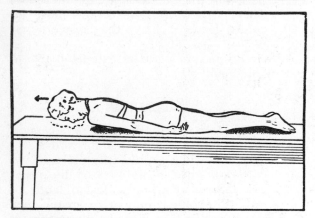

3. *Pronelying*
a. Arms at sides.
Raise head, rotate slowly to one side then lower to table, maintaining axial extension of the cervical spine. Repeat to other side (illustrated).
b. Head turned to one side resting on table, chin tucked in.
Raise the head, maintaining axial extension of the cervical spine, and turn slowly to other side, lower head to table and relax.
(Avoid pressure on hands or elbows).

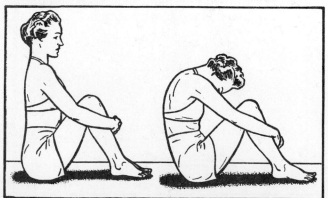

4. *Hooksitting,* hands clasped around knees.
Relax spine into a C curve and allow the head to drop down toward the knees.
Straighten the back, beginning with extension of the thoracic spine, then axial extension of the cervical spine.

ALIGNMENT OF CERVICAL SPINE

BASIC EXERCISES

5. *Cross sitting,* hands on lap, lumbar and thoracic spine straight.
a. Let the head fall forward on the chest. Return slowly to vertical position with axial extension of neck.
b. Let the head fall forward, then backward slowly, through as great a range as possible, allowing gravity to lengthen the neck muscles.
c. Let the head fall forward, then flex laterally (do not rotate the head but keep the face forward). Drop the head back, and then to the other side.
Continue head circling slowly, emphasizing muscle relaxation (Illustrated).

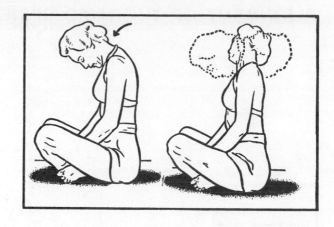

6. *Cross sitting,* head dropped forward, fingers interlaced behind head.
Move head up and back into a position of good axial extension, pushing against moderate resistance given by the hands.
After a series of head motions, lower arms slowly to the sides, maintaining the corrected position of the spine and head.

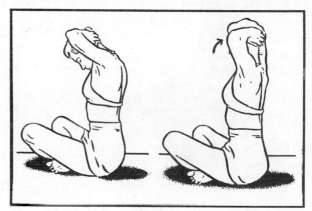

7. *Standing,* fingers interlaced above head, lumbar and thoracic spine straight.
a. Push the head upward toward the hands and practice walking, emphasizing axial extension of the cervical spine. Hold elbows back but avoid hyperextension of the lumbar spine.
b. Keep the arms at sides while walking, emphasizing the position of the head and spine.

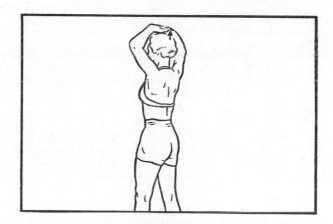

8. *Sitting in Sayre sling suspension.*
a. Pull down on the pulley rope to straighten cervical spine with traction. Release pull slowly attempting to maintain position.
b. Add neck rotation with moderate traction (illustrated) then release pull, maintaining position. (The sling should be carefully adjusted to head position.)
Increased axial extension can be obtained by sitting slightly behind the overhead pulley. The standing position may also be used.

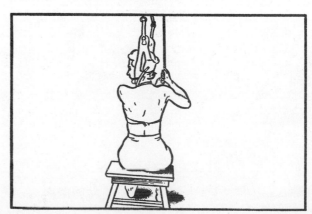

ALIGNMENT OF THORACIC SPINE AND SHOULDER GIRDLE

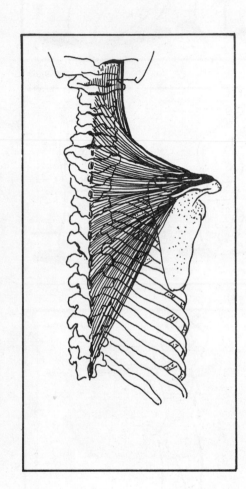

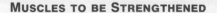

MUSCLES TO BE STRENGTHENED

SCAPULAR ADDUCTORS AND ROTATORS

Trapezius (Upper Fibers, Page 63)
Trapezius (Middle Fibers)

Origin: Spinous processes of the seventh cervical and upper thoracic vertebrae.

Insertion: Medial margin of the acromion and superior lip posterior border of scapula.

Trapezius (Lower Fibers)

Origin: Superior spine of the scapula, inferior thoracic vertebra, and supraspinal ligament.

Insertion: Aponeurosis to tubercle at apex of smooth triangular surface of scapula.

The three main divisions of the trapezius play varied roles in body alignment. The *upper fibers,* attaching to the clavicle, aid in suspending the shoulder girdle on the thorax. The supportive and rotary role of the upper part of the muscle changes as the position of the scapula changes during arm elevation. In the standing, resting position, the muscle is entirely supportive. With the last 35 degrees of elevation, the angle of action of the muscle changes, so that its force is equally divided between the supportive and the rotary roles. From 35 to 140 degrees, the muscle is increasingly more effective as a rotator.

The *middle fibers* pull directly in line with scapular adduction and help to keep the scapula from slipping laterally around the thorax when the arms are elevated. Weakness in this portion allows the scapula to assume an abducted position on the posterior chest wall.

The *lower fibers* of the trapezius assist with upward rotation of the scapula, which accompanies arm elevation. When the trunk is flexed even slightly, the arms cannot be supported overhead without the stabilizing force of this part of the muscle.

ALIGNMENT OF THORACIC SPINE AND SHOULDER GIRDLE

MUSCLES TO BE STRENGTHENED

Rhomboid Major and Minor

Origin: Spinous processes of the seventh cervical and first five thoracic vertebrae.

Insertion: Medial border of the scapula, from base of spine to inferior angle.

These muscles help to control the motions of the scapulae associated with arm movements. They are strong downward rotators of the scapulae, and their stabilizing action is particularly important during arm extension and hyperextension.

While the scapulae are suspended on the posterior thoracic wall by the upper trapezius, levator scapulae, and rhomboid muscles, they are held against the ribs by these and other scapular muscles, mainly the serratus anterior, middle and lower trapezius, and pectoralis minor.

As the scapulae rest against the upper posterior thoracic wall, their alignment depends largely upon the curve of the adjacent spine and the shape of the rib cage. If there is malalignment of either, exercise for scapular adduction will be of little value without an attempt to straighten the spine and flatten the thorax.

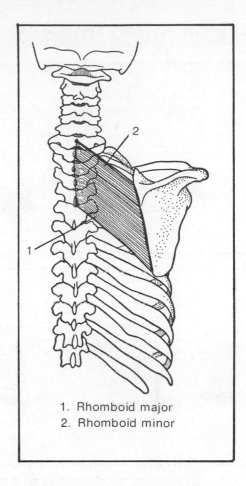

1. Rhomboid major
2. Rhomboid minor

LATERAL ROTATORS OF THE SHOULDER

Infraspinatus

Origin: Medial two thirds of the infraspinatus fossa.

Insertion: Middle impression on the greater tubercle of humerus.

Teres Minor

Origin: Cranial two thirds of the axillary border of the scapula on the dorsal surface.

Insertion: Most inferior of three impressions on the greater tubercle of the humerus and the area just distal to it, uniting with the posterior portion of the capsule of the shoulder joint.

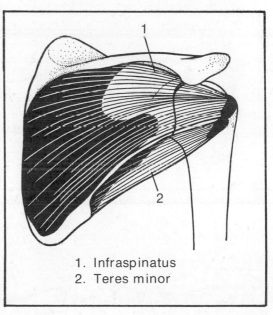

1. Infraspinatus
2. Teres minor

PRECAUTION

In exercises for the thoracic area of the spine and the shoulder girdle, contraction of the gluteal and abdominal musculature should be utilized to control the alignment of the pelvic segment and to prevent hyperextension of the lumbar spine.

ALIGNMENT OF THORACIC SPINE AND SHOULDER GIRDLE

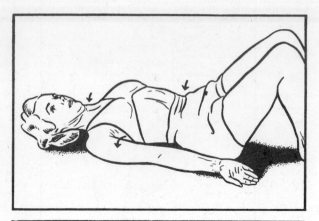

BASIC EXERCISES

1. *Hooklying,* arms at sides in complete medial rotation.
a. Flatten the lumbar and cervical spine against the table.
Rotate the arms laterally and adduct the scapulae. Hold, then relax and return to the starting position.
b. Make fists and flex elbows. Keeping elbows close to the sides, adduct the scapulae, reaching thumbs toward the table.

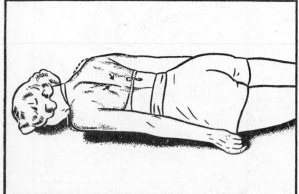

2. *Pronelying,* arms at sides.
Adduct the scapulae and pull downward toward the pelvis. Relax and return slowly to position.

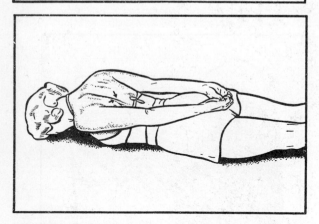

3. *Pronelying,* hands clasped behind pelvis.
a. Adduct the scapulae strongly. Relax and return to position.
b. Hold adducted position as hands are unclasped and returned to sides, then relax the scapular adductors.

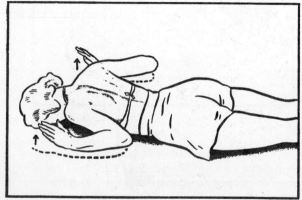

4. *Pronelying,* arms in reverse T, forehead resting on table.
Adduct the scapulae and elevate the arms, maintaining a position of 90 degrees at the shoulders and elbows. Keep the elbows and wrists parallel to the table. Return slowly to position.

ALIGNMENT OF THORACIC SPINE AND SHOULDER GIRDLE

BASIC EXERCISES

5. *Pronelying,* arms abducted, forehead resting on table.
Raise both arms as high as possible, keeping the head in position without lifting the chest from the table.
If the lumbar spine tends to hyperextend, have the subject begin with a pelvic tilt or place a pad under the abdomen at the level of the anterior superior iliac spine.

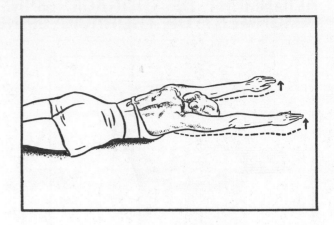

6. *Pronelying,* elbows completely flexed and held to the sides, with the forehead resting on the table.
Raise the flexed arms, extend both arms overhead, keeping the hands as high as the elbows: return the arms to the flexed position and lower to the table.

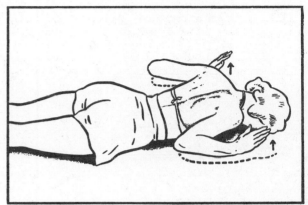

7. *Cross sitting*
Raise the arms to shoulder level, with the elbows flexed to a right angle and the forearms horizontal, palms facing.
Externally rotate the arms until the forearms are vertical, at the same time adducting the scapulae strongly. Maintain the scapular adduction and lower the arms to the sides.
(Extension of the spine should be maintained throughout the exercise).

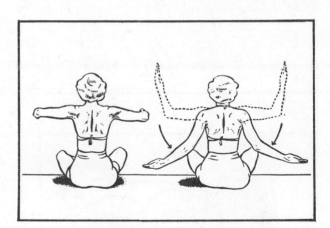

8. *Cross sitting,* arms at sides.
a. Circle one shoulder forward, up, back, and down, letting the arms hang free. Keep the thorax from turning with the movement.
b. Alternate circling of the right and left shoulders in a figure-of-eight pattern. Emphasize the backward and downward phase of the circle.
c. Repeat in a reverse direction, always stressing the phase of the circle in which the scapula is adducted and drawn downward.

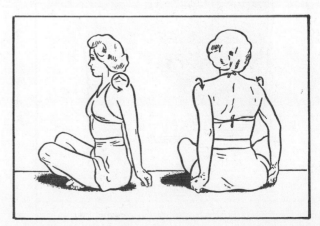

ALIGNMENT OF THORACIC SPINE AND SHOULDER GIRDLE

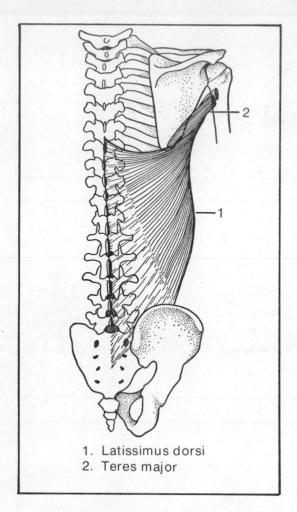

1. Latissimus dorsi
2. Teres major

MUSCLES THAT MAY NEED STRETCHING

SHOULDER ADDUCTORS AND MEDIAL ROTATORS

Latissimus Dorsi

Origin: Spinous processes of lower six thoracic, lumbar, and sacral vertebrae via the lumbodorsal fascia, posterior iliac crest and caudal three or four ribs.

Insertion: Bottom of the intertubercular groove of humerus.

Teres Major

Origin: Dorsal surface of the inferior angle of the scapula.

Insertion: Crest below the lesser tuberosity of the humerus (posterior to the latissimus dorsi).

In the subject with habitual round shoulders (abducted scapulae), the muscles between the stretching procedures the scapula must be firmly stabilized as the arm is elevated or laterally rotated.

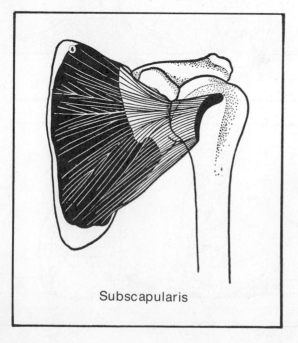

Subscapularis

Subscapularis

Origin: Medial two thirds of the costal surface of the scapula. Inferior two thirds of the groove on the axillary border of the scapula.

Insertion: Lesser tubercle of the humerus and the ventral portion of the capsule of the shoulder joint.

ALIGNMENT OF THORACIC SPINE AND SHOULDER GIRDLE

MUSCLES THAT MAY NEED STRETCHING

SHOULDER ADDUCTORS AND MEDIAL ROTATORS

Pectoralis Major

Origin: Medial one third of the clavicle, anterior surface of the sternum and cartilages of the first six or seven ribs.

Insertion: Crest below the greater tubercle of the humerus.

This extensive muscle is often shortened in persons with relaxed posture, hollow chest, and round shoulders. Outward rotation of the humerus increases the tension on this muscle. When the arm is placed above a right angle, greater stretch is applied to the sternal fibers. In order to obtain an effective stretch of this muscle, the thorax must be fixed.

Pectoralis Minor (Not Illustrated)

Origin: Third, fourth and fifth ribs.

Insertion: Coracoid process of the humerus.

Shortening of this muscle is associated with forward tilting of the scapula and protrusion of the inferior angle.

PRECAUTION

In stretching procedures for the shoulder adductors and medial rotators, the scapulae must be firmly stabilized.

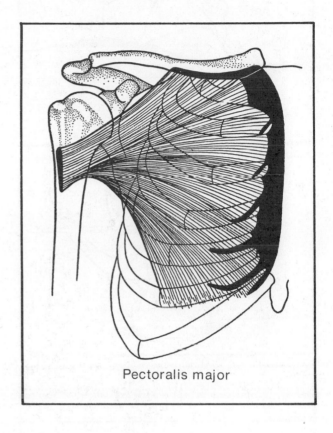

Pectoralis major

ALIGNMENT OF THORACIC SPINE AND SHOULDER GIRDLE

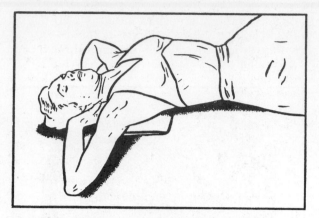

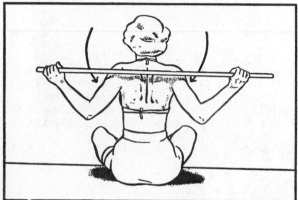

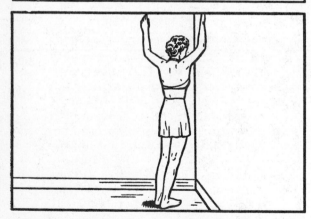

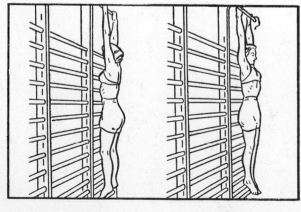

EXERCISES FOR STRETCHING SHOULDER ADDUCTORS AND MEDIAL ROTATORS

1. *Hooklying,* with a pad or small folded towel placed under the midthoracic area.
a. Hands behind neck.
Adduct scapulae and force elbows down toward table (illustrated).
b. Arms completely abducted.
Force elbows and forearms downward toward table. Keep spine flat.
c. Arms completely abducted.
Flex hips and bring knees as close as possible to chest.

2. *Cross sitting* on table.
a. Grasp the ends of a wand and extend the arms overhead. Bring the wand down posterior to the shoulders, flexing the elbows. Maintain axial extension of the neck and extension of the thoracic spine.
b. Bring the wand down behind the trunk and then return it overhead.
(Many variations of wand exercises are possible. Pectoral muscle length may be increased by moving the hands closer together on the wand.)

3. *Standing,* facing one corner of the room. Arms in reverse T position or slightly above 90 degrees of abduction. Rest foreams against the wall on either side of the corner and lean forward from ankles. Keep spine, hips, and knees straight. The heels should remain in contact with the floor to assist in maintaining vertical position of the body.
(A narrow open doorway may be used. Forearms are placed on each side of uprights.)

4. *Standing*
a. Face stall bars, grasp cross bar with arms in full abduction, flex knees slowly for stretch.
b. Place back to stall bars and repeat exercise.
c. Step on low bar and grasp cross bar overhead. Take partial or full weight on arms as indicated (illustrated).
d. Step on low bar, turn and grasp bar overhead. Adjust weight (illustrated).

THE THORACIC SPINE AND RIB CAGE

MECHANICS OF RESPIRATION

CONTOUR AND MOVEMENTS OF THE THORAX

The rib cage is so arranged that with inspiration the thorax increases in size in three directions—in width, depth, and vertical dimension. The upper ribs move primarily in an up and down direction, while the lower ribs move inward and outward, traveling in a transverse plane.

Grant compares the second to seventh rib arches to inverted bucket handles, each of which is attached to the vertebral column posteriorly and to the sternum in front. The sternal end is lower than the vertebral. These six ribs increase in length, lateral projection, and obliquity from the second rib downward. On inspiration, they rotate about their vertebral joints so that their middle parts rise, and at the same time the sternum is pushed anteriorly and upward. During ordinary respiration, the first rib remains at rest.

The eighth, ninth and tenth ribs, attached anteriorly only by cartilage, move outward during inspiration like a pair of opening calipers, and the subcostal angle widens. It seems paradoxical that the dome-shaped diaphragm muscle, situated within the thorax, can cause the ribs to which it is attached to move in an outward direction. According to Grant, this results from tension of the abdominal muscles

which forces the contents of the upper abdominal cavity to move laterally as the diaphragm pushes downward in inspiration. By this means the distal ribs are carried sideward.

Gardner et al. describe the movement of the ribs as the so-called "pump-handle" and "bucket-handle" movements. In the former, the upper ribs primarily move about a side-to-side axis at the costovertebral joints, resulting in raising and lowering the sternal end of the ribs. The latter, the "bucket-handle" movement, takes place chiefly at the costotransverse joints of the lower ribs about a front-to-back axis, leading to depression or elevation of the middle of the ribs (Fig. 17).

Davis and Troup state that a forward, upward, or lateral movement of the bony cage of only a few millimeters is sufficient to increase the volume of the thoracic cage by almost one half liter. This is the usual volume of air that enters and leaves the lungs during quiet breathing.

Gardner et al. note that the range of movement at each of the thoracic joints is small, but any disorder that reduces their mobility hampers respiration.

Steindler emphasizes the importance of the elastic resistance with which the ribs oppose their anchorage at either end. This is such that the thorax would spring open if it were cut longitudinally on either side. The elastic resistance of the ribs increases or decreases in inspiration or expiration as the ribs bend and straighten. The neutral level of this intrinsic equilibrium is somewhere between full inspiration and full expiration, "somewhat on the side of inspiration," according to Steindler. Thus muscular effort is required both for expansion and full contraction of the thorax.

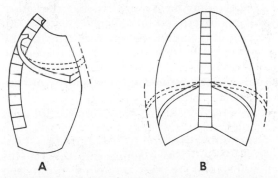

A   **B**

Figure 17. Representation of certain movements of the ribs. In lateral view, *A*, when the upper ribs are elevated, the anteroposterior diameter of the thorax is increased ("pump-handle" movement). In posterior view, *B*, the lower ribs move laterally when they are elevated, and the transverse diameter of the thorax is increased ("bucket-handle" movement). (From Gardner, E., Gray, D. L., and O'Rahilly, R., Anatomy. 4th ed., Philadelphia, W. B. Saunders Co., 1975.)

COMBINED MOTIONS OF THE THORACIC SPINE AND RIB CAGE

Motions of the thoracic spine and of the rib cage are interdependent. When the spine is flexed, the ribs are depressed, and their excursion is limited. When the thoracic spine is extended, the ribs become elevated, and the chest wall moves laterally, anteriorly, and upward. Thus, the posture patient with "fatigue slump" characterized by habitual round back, hollow chest, and abducted scapulae may be expected to have limitation in the flexibility of the thorax. Fortunately, there are many muscles concerned with thoracic, spinal, and humeral movement which may be activated to expand the rib cage and help in restoring its normal contour and mobility.

It should be noted that the position of the head and neck is important in the alignment of the rib cage. With a forward head and neck, the ventral scalene muscles, raising the first and second ribs, are put on a slack. With the correction of the alignment of the head and neck (axial extension, pages 48, 49 and 50), these muscles are in position to fix the upper ribs and thus assist the elevation of the chest wall.

FUNCTION OF MUSCLES OF RESPIRATION

The diaphragm is the principal muscle of respiration. In quiet respiration, it may act alone or there may be a slight rhythmic activity in the scalenus anterior and medius and in the intercostals. Quiet expiration is relatively passive, owing to the elastic recoil of the lungs and the elasticity of the ligaments and cartilages that hold the ribs and other structures in place. Electromyography has demonstrated some activity in the interosseus internal intercostals of the seventh to tenth interspaces.

In deep inspiration, the action of the primary muscles is increased. Assistance in raising the ribs is given by the sternocleidomastoids and the scaleni. Other muscles attached to the rib cage may become active to expand the thorax according to the degree of need.

In forced expiration, the muscles of the abdominal wall, particularly the oblique and transverse portions, contract to force the diaphragm upward and the ribs downward and medially. The quadratus lumborum also may draw the ribs downward, with assistance from other muscles attached to the thorax.

The level of the diaphragm varies with the posture of the individual, being highest in the supine position, lower in the standing position, and lowest in the sitting position. This explains why the person with severe shortness of breath is most comfortable in the sitting position, where a minimum excursion of the diaphragm is required.

CHANGES IN RESPIRATION WITH AGE

Because the ribs are horizontal at birth, or in a position of full inspiration, breathing must be carried out during the early period of life by the piston-like excursion of the diaphragm (abdominal breathing). As the child grows, the chest gradually flattens anteroposteriorly and the ribs become oblique. As a result, the excursion of the ribs in elevation and lowering causes the thoracic capacity and hence the lung area to expand and contract (thoracic breathing).

In the adult, breathing is a combination of both abdominal and thoracic breathing, although any given individual may breath predominantly one way or the other. The type of breathing can be controlled voluntarily.

SELECTION OF EXERCISES

Exercise for thoracic surgery patients given both pre- and postoperatively has become an important part of the physical therapist's armamentarium. Formation of scar tissue following any type of surgery, together with the tendency of the patient to guard the affected area against painful movement, may result in permanent immobilization and severe structural and functional deformity. During World War II, techniques in exercise therapy for chest surgery cases were developed which require fine localization of motion in specific areas of the thorax.

A scoliotic patient with a primary thoracic curve may have a greatly distorted chest wall. As discussed on page 17, the diagonal diameter is increased on the side of the convexity of the curve and decreased on the opposite side. On the convex side, the thoracic cage bulges out posteriorly and appears flat anteriorly. Mobility here can be encouraged by the patient himself through manual means. He may exert pressure with one hand against the ribs that are flared anteriorly, and by placing the tips of his fingers beneath the opposite, depressed ribs at the subcostal angle, he may pull them outward and upward with the other hand. In other words, with inspiration the hand on the concave side pushes the flared ribs inward while that on the opposite side lifts and spreads the depressed ribs.

The problem of the asthmatic individual is quite different from that of the person with a hollow chest and depressed rib cage. He is troubled by overexpansion of the chest and has difficulty in expiration. If his asthma has been of sufficient severity and long standing, the thorax may adapt permanently to its inflated shape and become a "barrel chest." Such persons must practice control of the expiratory phase of breathing and develop the muscles involved with compression of the thorax.

Gravity favors expiration, particularly in the erect or prone positions. In the supine position, the use of a large pillow beneath the head and upper spine causes rounding of the thoracic spine and limits excursion of the rib cage and lungs. In a sidelying position, the dome of the diaphragm on the lower side makes a greater excursion than that on the upper side.

MUSCLES OF RESPIRATION

PRIMARY MUSCLES OF INSPIRATION

Diaphragm (not illustrated)

Origin: Sternal part from the xiphoid process, costal part from inner surface cartilages and adjacent portion of last six ribs, and lumbar part from the lumbar vertebrae.

Insertion: Central tendon, somewhat closer to the ventral than the dorsal part.

External Intercostals (11 in number, not illustrated)

These extend from the tubercles of the ribs dorsally to the cartilages of the ribs ventrally, and end in thin membranes continued toward the sternum.

Origin of each: Caudal border of a rib.

Insertion of each: Cranial border of the rib below.

The fibers are oblique (same direction as the external oblique abdominal muscle, page 50).

PRIMARY MUSCLES OF EXPIRATION

Internal Intercostals (11 in number, not illustrated)

In quiet expiration there is some activity in the internal intercostals.

These muscles commence at the sternum in the interspace between the cartilages of the true ribs and at the ventral extremities of the false ribs. They extend dorsalward as far as the angles of the ribs, then by thin aponeuroses to the ventral column.

Origin: Ridge on the inner surface of a rib and the corresponding costal cartilage.

Insertion: Cranial border of rib below.

The fibers are oblique (same direction as the internal oblique abdominal muscle, page 50).

The anterolateral external abdominal muscles are the important muscles of forced expiration. These muscles are the rectus abdominis (page 50), external and internal obliques (page 50) and the transversus abdominis (not illustrated).

THORACIC SPINE AND RIB CAGE

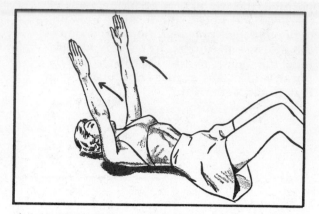

1. *Hooklying*, arms at sides, cervical and lumbar spine flat.
   a. Flex one arm to vertical, at the same time attempting to expand the chest on that side with a deep breath.
   Exhale as the arm is lowered slowly.
   Repeat on the opposite side.
   b. Flex both arms to vertical and then overhead, lifting rib cage as much as possible.
   Exhale as arms are lowered slowly to sides (illustrated).

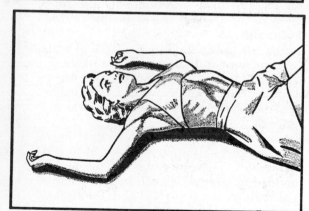

2. *Hooklying*, hands on lower sides of thorax and vertical to table.
   a. Inhale against mild pressure of hands downward and inward.
   b. Inhale against strong pressure of hands.
   Grasp with the fingers under costal extremities. Attempt to very gently pull rib cage upward and outward with fingertips to increase range of rib excursion.

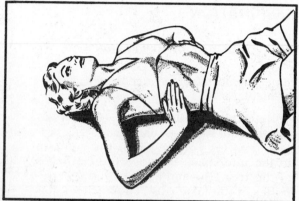

3. *Hooklying*, arms at sides.
   a. Breathe in, allowing the abdomen to rise; transfer the air to the upper chest with the throat closed. Exhale slowly.
   b. Breathe in, allowing the chest to rise moderately. Hold the chest position and exhale by contracting the abdominal muscles. Lift ribs a little higher with next breath, hold rib position, then exhale. Repeat until the thorax is fully elevated and no more air can be passed into upper chest. Relax and repeat.

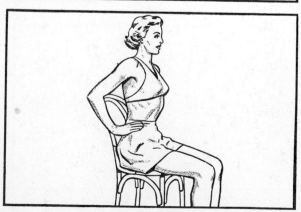

4. *Sitting*, hands on hips.
   a. Breathe deeply, pushing chest up and forward, force downward with hands on hips. Hold chest position and exhale, contracting abdominal muscles. Relax.
   b. Repeat, using a small series of inspirations until the thorax is completely expanded. (Standing position may also be used).

THORACIC SPINE AND RIB CAGE

BASIC EXERCISES EMPHASIZING EXPIRATION

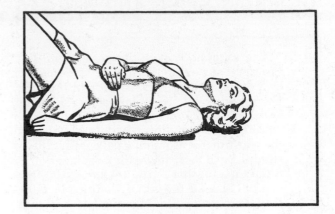

1. *Hooklying,* one hand on abdomen.
Breathe out slowly and completely by contracting abdominal muscles. (Feel the depression of the abdominal wall as it sinks.)
Breathe in gently and repeat.

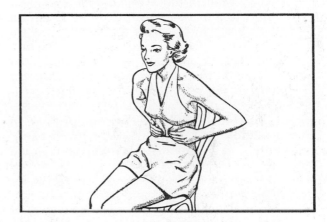

2. *Sitting,* hands on lower ribs, fingers
   pointing forward.
Breathe out by contracting the abdominal muscles strongly. (Feel the compression of the lower rib cage.) Exert pressure with the hands at the end of exhalation to expel as much air as possible. Relax and repeat.

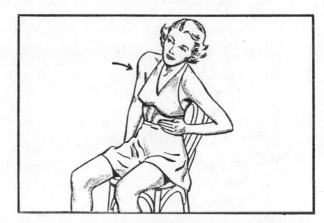

3. *Sitting,* one hand over lower ribs on one
   side of thorax, fingers pointing forward.
During strong expiration by contraction of abdominal muscles, flex trunk laterally and forward toward the hand and exert strong manual pressure to increase the compression of the ribs on that side. Repeat on opposite side.

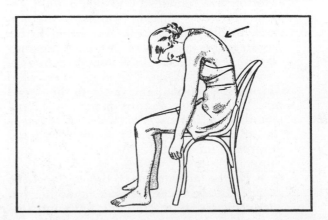

4. *Sitting,* arms relaxed at sides.
Allow the upper trunk to fall forward with
   flexion of cervical and thoracic spine.
Contract the abdominal muscles strongly,
   compressing the lower ribs.
Return to position, breathing in moderately
   and freely.
(In all exercises, the expiration phase
   should be made to last as long as possible.)

THE LOWER EXTREMITY

The alignment of the lower extremity in the upright position, whether stationary or in motion, is basic to posture and function. Deviations such as hyperextended knees, knock knees, bowlegs, and tibial torsion were previously described in relation to the posture evaluation (pages 14, 20). It should be noted, in further explanation of tibial torsion, that a true torsion of the tibia is a twisting of the tibial shaft itself. However, the term "tibial torsion" as it is commonly used in the evaluation of alignment refers to a marked rotation of the femur on the tibia, which causes the patellae to face somewhat medially and is part of the normal locking mechanism. Controlled contraction of the lateral rotators of the hip can help in the restoration of a balanced position.

Shortened muscles that are present in variations in alignment of the lower extremities are commonly related to medial rotation and adduction of the thighs. However, in the person who has been bed-ridden for long periods of time, and often in the geriatric patient, the lateral rotators may be at fault. Exercises for stretching tight hip flexors have been omitted from this section, for, although they are frequently found to be shortened, they primarily affect pelvic tilt rather than leg position and therefore were considered with the pelvic segment and lumbar spine (pages 60, 61).

FOOT PLACEMENT

The placement of the feet during standing and walking is dependent upon the position of the lower extremity and may be controlled at the hip joint. Among others, Morton has demonstrated that a mild degree of out-toe walking is found in the normal, healthy individual. According to his studies, the position of greatest efficiency for the feet is between 30 and 40 degrees of out-toe for standing. The angle is reduced during locomotion, varying with the speed and consequent requirements for lateral stability. It is between 14 and 20 degrees in ordinary walking, and the feet naturally approach the parallel position only in running.

Both the alignment of the leg and the longitudinal arch of the foot should be considered in determining the optimum foot position recommended for each individual, insofar as this can be controlled. A marked out-toe angle should be avoided in those cases with a tendency toward foot pronation or flat foot. On the other hand, near parallel placement of the feet should not be forced on the person whose patellae will be markedly faced medially, resulting in an awkward stance and gait.

ARCHES OF THE FOOT

The bones of the medial longitudinal section of the foot, consisting of the three medial digits, their metatarsals, and the three cuneiform bones, the navicular and talus, together with the calcaneus form a medial longitudinal spring or arch. Viewed from the medial aspect, the posterior pillar of the arch rests on the medial tubercle of the calcaneus, and the anterior pillar rests on the sesamoid bones beneath the head of the first metatarsal. At the summit of the arch is the talus, resting above and between the sustentaculum tali and the navicular bone.

The plantar calcaneonavicular ligament and the tibialis posterior muscle serve to support the long arch of the foot, the apex of which lies at the junction of its posterior one third and anterior thirds (Fig. 18).

The bones of the lateral section of the foot, forming the lateral arch, are the calcaneus, cuboid, and lateral two metatarsals and digits.

In addition to the longitudinal arches a series of transverse arches are described,

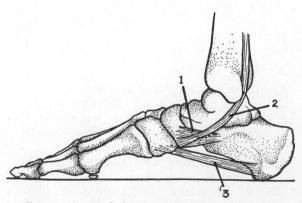

Figure 18. Medial view of the foot, with major structures which support the long arch. *1,* Calcaneonavicular ligament; *2,* tibialis posterior muscle; *3,* long plantar ligament.

which present a half dome so that when the medial borders of the feet are approximated a complete tarsal dome is formed. The weight is transferred to the floor through the region of the metatarsal heads and to some degree the lateral border of the foot.

WEIGHT-BEARING FORCES

A number of investigators, including Abramsen, Elftman, Morton, and Jones measured weight-bearing forces and demonstrated that each of the five metatarsal heads bears a definite portion of the body load. Morton may be cited as an exponent of the view that weight is supported by the entire anterior metatarsal area. He found, by means of pressure measurements, that the weight is normally distributed on the heel and forefoot equally. Anteriorly, pressure is carried on each metatarsal head, with the first supporting a double share so that the ratio is 2:1:1:1:1. Thus, the space beneath the foot may be considered a series of arches extending between the calcaneal tubercles and each metatarsal head.

In studies on locomotion, Schwartz and Heath have measured various foot areas to determine the time and duration of stance and the force normally exerted on the metatarsal heads. They found that pressure on the third metatarsal head is considerably greater than that on the first or fifth, and the duration of weight bearing slightly longer.

On the basis of these investigations, there is no reason to view the foot as divided into two functional segments, medial and lateral, or to advocate an attempt to preserve a transverse metatarsal arch by voluntary effort during walking.

It should be pointed out that the height of the arch varies with each individual and that a simple depression of the longitudinal arch with balanced muscle control is not uncommon and is not pathological. It may represent a strong and stable foot. Discomfort or pain, particularly after standing for a period of time, are symptoms that are of importance in differentiating the abnormal from the normal arch.

MUSCLES CONTROLLING THE FOOT

In static planovalgus, or flatfoot, the long arch is flattened out and rolled toward the medial border of the foot, which assumes a convex appearance. Steindler pointed out that the principal muscle supporting the longitudinal arch is the tibialis posterior. It is assisted by the great toe flexor, as well as by the flexor digitorum longus. The posterior tibial inserts into the tuberosity of the navicular and sends fibrous expansions to the sustentaculum tali posteriorly, and forward and laterally to the three cuneiforms, the cuboid, and bases of the second, third, and fourth metatarsals (page 90). Thus, its location indicates that it is of particular importance in the muscular control of the long foot arch. Since the tendon of the flexor hallucis longus passes beneath the sustentaculum tali, it helps to hold up this shelf, upon which the talus rests. Proper elevation of this point serves to keep the calcaneus from tipping medially into a position of eversion, predisposing to foot pronation.

The transverse arches are strengthened by the peroneus longus, the tendon of which stretches between the piers of the arches.

It has been reported by Lowman that the tibialis anterior muscle may be hypertrophied at the same time that the long arch is completely flat. According to this interpretation, the pull of this muscle comes too far forward on the foot to help maintain the position of the long arch. Since it elevates (and supinates) the forepart of the foot, raising of this section rather than of the midarch bones by the tibialis anterior may even be harmful in second and third degree flatfoot.

In the standing position, the muscles of the foot are relaxed, which places the stress on the plantar ligaments for support of the longitudinal arch. On movement, the muscles must react strongly to maintain the balance of the foot and to protect the ligamentous structures as well as to propel the body forward. It has been noted that when the body is raised on the ball of one foot, ths stress on the arch is increased four times.

EXERCISE PROGRAM

A proper balance between the muscles controlling the hip and the knee is essential to good alignment and function of the lower extremity, and exercises are presented to assist the individual to attain this goal. All of these muscles affect the stability of the foot.

In the control of foot position, however,

the muscles that pronate and supinate the feet require particular attention. Since the common tendency is toward pronation, this should be identified and, when present, exercise for the medial muscles instituted. In walking, placing the whole foot on the floor without deviation either medially or laterally should be emphasized.

For correction of hammer toes, the pull of the interossei and lumbricales is most effective. Exercise of these and other small intrinsic muscles of the forefoot increases the mobility and control of the foot in walking. The toes, which are often neglected and which play little part in the walking pattern, should be used for gripping and pushing off at the end of the supporting phase of the step. Exercises such as picking up marbles with the toes and toe curling around a towel may be beneficial only if flexion occurs at the metatarsophalangeal joints as well as at the interphalangeal joints.

An exercise program can increase the mobility of the foot, which too often is used as a stiff, inflexible part. Manual stretching may be a necessary component for mobilizing the foot joints. Fine movements, such as toe abduction or flexion at the metatarsophalangeal joints, can assist the person in gaining control of the various areas of the foot and in becoming conscious of their use in walking. Finally, the development of a kinesthetic sense of position and control is essential in improving the alignment of the foot and in carrying out its two important functions: 1) to support the weight of the body in standing and progression and 2) to act as a lever in propelling the body forward.

FOR NOTES:

ALIGNMENT OF THE LOWER EXTREMITY

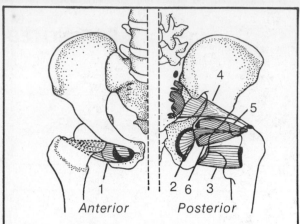

Anterior	*Posterior*

1. Obturator externus   4. Piriformis
2. Obturator internus   5. Gemellus superior
3. Quadratus femoris   6. Gemellus inferior

MUSCLES TO BE STRENGTHENED

HIP ROTATORS

Lateral Rotators

Origin: Seven muscles are prime movers in hip lateral rotation, five of which arise from the pubis, ischium, or both, one from the sacrum, and one, the gluteus maximus (page 84) from the iliac crest, sacrum and coccyx; one muscle, the piriformis, crosses the sacroiliac articulation.

Insertion: All insert into the trochanteric fossa, greater trochanter, linea quadrata, gluteal tuberosity, or iliotibial band.

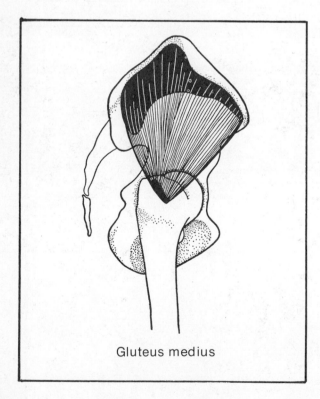

Gluteus medius

HIP ABDUCTOR

Gluteus Medius

Origin: The outer surface of the ilium, between the iliac crest and the posterior gluteal line dorsally and the anterior gluteal line ventrally.

Insertion: An oblique ridge on the lateral surface of the greater trochanter.

The primary function of the hip abductor is to stabilize the pelvis over the supporting leg during unilateral weight bearing.* Weakness in this muscle causes either a shift in the pelvis toward the supported side or an exaggerated drop on the unsupported side (Trendelenburg sign).

---

* For variations in abductor gait, see *Muscle Testing*.

ALIGNMENT OF THE LOWER EXTREMITY

EXERCISES FOR LATERAL ROTATORS OF HIP

1. *Prone lying,* arms in reverse T or underneath head, big toes together and heels apart.
Bring the heels together with a strong contraction of the hip lateral rotators. Relax slowly and completely.

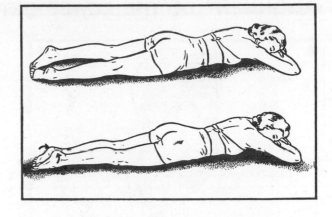

2. *Standing,* feet slightly apart and parallel, keeping metatarsal heads firmly on floor.
Flex the knees slightly, strongly rotate the thighs laterally, then extend the knees (avoid hyperextension). Finish the movement with the thighs in a neutral position of rotation.
(External rotation of the thigh with the foot fixed raises the longitudinal arch of the foot and also helps correct tibial torsion.)

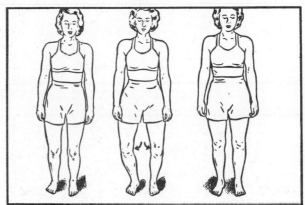

EXERCISES FOR ABDUCTORS OF THE HIP

1. *Sidelying,* underneath leg flexed for balance.
a. Abduct the leg through a range of approximately 45 degrees without rotation.
Return slowly to starting position.
b. Abduct and hold for several counts before lowering slowly.

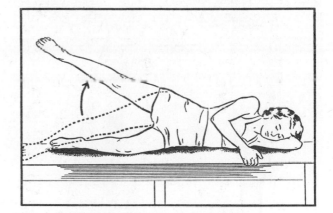

2. *Standing,* holding back of chair lightly for balance.
a. Lift one foot clear of the floor and allow the pelvis to drop on that side.
Elevate the pelvis on the unsupported side by a strong contraction of the hip abductors on the side of the supporting extremity. (In the illustration, hip abductors are contracting to raise and to control lowering of the left side of the pelvis.)
b. Shift weight in place, without support for balance. Walk, with emphasis on abductor function in the control of the pelvis.

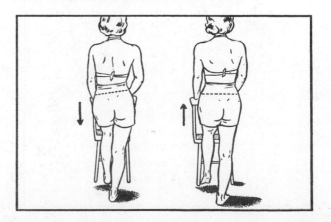

ALIGNMENT OF THE LOWER EXTREMITY

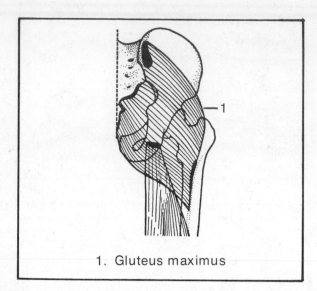

1. Gluteus maximus

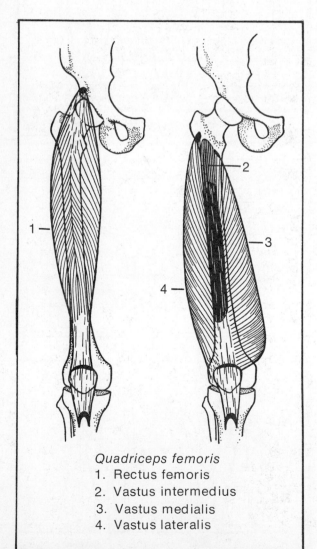

Quadriceps femoris
1. Rectus femoris
2. Vastus intermedius
3. Vastus medialis
4. Vastus lateralis

MUSCLES TO BE STRENGTHENED

HIP EXTENSOR

Gluteus Maximus

Origin and insertion (see page 51).

In addition to extension of the hip, this muscle is in a position to assist with posterior rotation of the pelvis (previously noted) and to correct excessive medial rotation of the thigh associated with "tibial torsion" (page 20).

KNEE EXTENSOR

Quadriceps Femoris

Rectus Femoris

Origin: Anterior inferior spine of ilium and reflected head from groove above brim of acetabulum.
Insertion: Proximal border of patella.

Vastus Intermedius

Origin: Upper two thirds of anterior and lateral surfaces of femoral shaft.
Insertion: Base of patella.

Vastus Medialis

Origin: Distal part of intertrochanteric line, linea aspera, and medial supracondylar ridge.
Insertion: Medial border of patella and quadriceps femoris tendon.

Vastus Lateralis

Origin: Proximal part of intertrochanteric line, borders of greater trochanter, and lateral lip of linea aspera.
Insertion: Base and lateral border of patella and quadriceps femoris tendon

The knee extensor muscles are important antigravity muscles in walking but are not required in standing, since the gravity line of the body falls anterior to the knee joint axis. The transverse direction of the distal fibers of the vastus medialis is a factor in preventing the patella from slipping laterally near the end of the extension.

The most superficial of the quadriceps group, the rectus femoris, crosses the hip as well as the knee joint; thus the position of both joints must always be considered in an analysis of the function of this muscle.

ALIGNMENT OF THE LOWER EXTREMITY

EXERCISES FOR HIP EXTENSORS

1. *Prone lying*
Hyperextend one hip a few inches from the table with a strong contraction of the gluteus maximus. Return slowly to position and repeat with other leg.
(Lifting the leg more than a few inches from table results in hyperextension of the lumbar spine, as the hip motion is very limited. The knees may be flexed to increase the participation of the hamstrings; however, increased tension in the rectus femoris will further limit range of motion.)

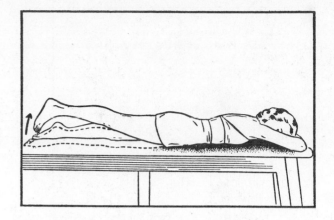

2. *Kneeling*, forehead resting on hands, spine straight, and thighs at right angle to table.
Extend one leg until it is in line with trunk. Return slowly to position and repeat to other side. Avoid lumbar hyperextension and rotation of trunk.
(This exercise is a good progression for the younger posture patient. Lack of balance, circulatory problems, or general debility will limit its usefulness.)

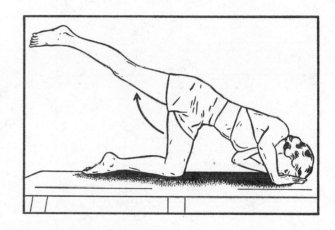

3. *Prone lying*, arms reverse T, hands grasping edge of table. Small pad or pillow under pelvis, legs over edge of table, toes touching floor, knees relaxed.
Extend both knees, then extend one hip to horizontal with knee straight. Lower leg slowly until foot contacts floor. Repeat with other leg. Relax knees. (Not illustrated).

EXERCISE FOR HIP AND KNEE EXTENSORS

1. *Standing*, with one foot on a low stool or stair.
a. Alternately extend the knee and hip of the forward foot to elevate the body, and then step down again (illustrated).
b. Increase height of stool as muscle strength improves (illustrated).
(Movement combines the use of hip and knee extensors. Shifting the trunk forward at the hips lengthens the hip extensors for greater participation in the lift and less strain on the quadriceps femoris and knee joint.)

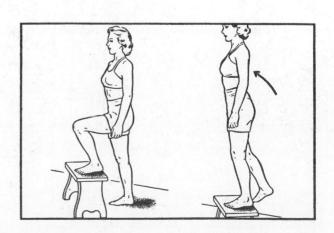

ALIGNMENT OF THE LOWER EXTREMITY

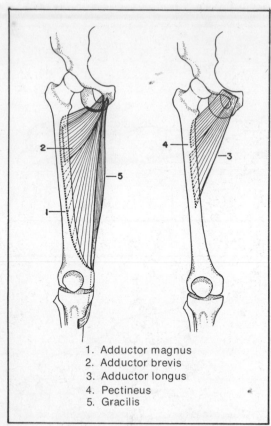

1. Adductor magnus
2. Adductor brevis
3. Adductor longus
4. Pectineus
5. Gracilis

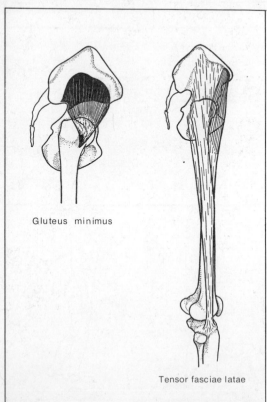

Gluteus minimus

Tensor fasciae latae

HIP ADDUCTORS

Adductor Magnus, Brevis, and Longus; Gracilis; and Pectineus

Origin: Superior and inferior rami of pubis and inferior ramus of ischium.

Insertion: Region of linea aspera and medial supracondylar line of femur.

The gracilis crosses the knee to insert on the proximal end of the tibia.

Shortening of the adductor group may be a limiting factor in the correction of knock knee. Since the upper fibers attach to the anterior portion of the pelvis, they are also in a position to oppose correction of an anterior pelvic tilt if they have become shortened.

HIP MEDIAL ROTATORS

Gluteus Minimus

Origin: Outer surface of ilium between anterior and inferior gluteal lines.

Insertion: Anterior surface of greater trochanter of femur.

Tensor Fasciae Latae

Origin: Anterior part of iliac crest.

Insertion: Iliotibial band at juncture of middle and upper thirds.

The tensor fasciae latae has attachments on the pelvis, femur, and tibia, and gives rise to some of the fibers of the short head of the biceps femoris and the vastus lateralis. Contracture of the iliotibial band complex results in knock knee, hip flexion, and abduction deformities. This means that with weight bearing, the pelvis tilts anteriorly and laterally, and is likely to be rotated in the horizontal plane. Pain as the result of stress on the low back structures can result.

HIP LATERAL ROTATORS

Obturators, Gemelli, Quadratus Femoris, and Piriformis

Origin and insertion: See page 82.
See discussion on page 83.

ALIGNMENT OF THE LOWER EXTREMITY

EXERCISE FOR STRETCHING HIP ADDUCTORS (AND HAMSTRINGS)

1. *Supine,* hips flexed, knees extended, hands underneath neck or in reverse T.
Abduct the legs as far as possible without lateral rotation. Hold. Flex knees to trunk then extend to starting position.
(Use mat if subject is uncomfortable on table.)

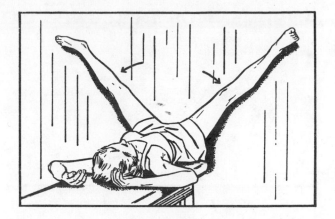

EXERCISES FOR STRETCHING HIP MEDIAL ROTATORS (AND ADDUCTORS)

1. *Sitting,* soles of feet together, trunk and head in good position, hands resting on knees.
Laterally rotate and abduct thighs. Hold and relax.
(The stretch may be decreased by placing the feet farther away from the trunk, or increased by pulling them back toward the pelvis.)

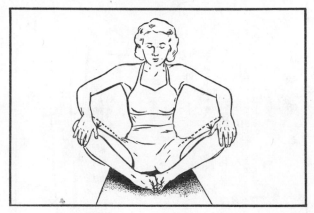

2. *Sitting,* soles of feet together, hands clasped around forefeet, or grasping ankles.
Flex the hips (keeping spine extended) through as great a range as possible. Hold, then return to position.

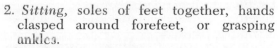

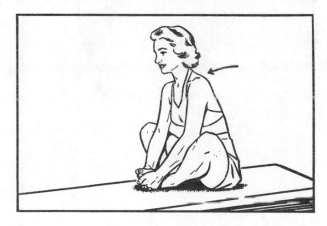

EXERCISE FOR STRETCHING HIP LATERAL ROTATORS

1. *Supine,* slight shoulder abduction and elbow flexion for stability.
a. Medially rotate the thigh (ankle dorsiflexed). Hold, then relax (illustrated).
b. Medially rotate both thighs. Hold, then relax.

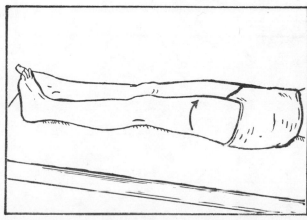

ALIGNMENT OF THE LOWER EXTREMITY

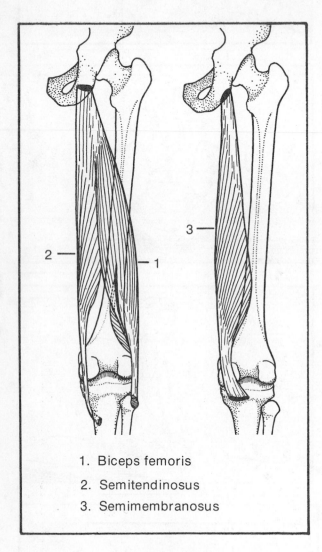

1. Biceps femoris
2. Semitendinosus
3. Semimembranosus

KNEE FLEXORS

Hamstrings

Biceps Femoris

Origin: Long head—ischial tuberosity.
Short head—lateral lip of linea aspera, lateral supracondylar line of femur.
Insertion: Both muscles, into head of fibula and lateral condyle of tibia.

Semitendinosus

Origin: Ischial tuberosity.
Insertion: Anteromedial surface of proximal end of tibia.

Semimembranosus

Origin: Ischial tuberosity.
Insertion: Posteromedial aspect of medial condyle of tibia.
The downward pull of the hamstring muscles is in a direct line to rotate the pelvis posteriorly. Since these muscles are attached far back on the ischial tuberosity, they have a good lever arm in this motion.
The tendons of these muscles cross behind the knee joint and help to prevent hyperextended knee in the weight-bearing position (see discussion on page 5).

ALIGNMENT OF THE LOWER EXTREMITY

EXERCISES FOR STRETCHING HAMSTRINGS

1. *Supine*, arms partially abducted or in a reverse T position.

Flex one hip with knee extended, attempting to increase range of motion. Keep opposite leg in complete extension on table. Do not allow the thigh to rotate.

(Dorsiflexion of the foot may be added; this helps maintain the knee in extension by the reverse pull of the gastrocnemius and soleus from their origins posterior to the knee joint.)

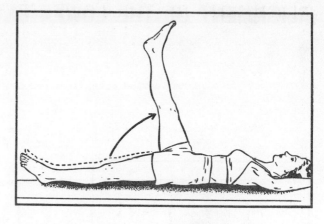

2. *Supine*, arms at sides.
a. Flex trunk and hips to a sitting position. Attempt to rotate pelvis anteriorly without flexion of thoracic spine or undue strain on lumbar extensors for isolation of hamstring stretch.
b. Abduct legs, rotate trunk to one side, and rotate pelvis anteriorly. Then rotate to other side to emphasize single hamstring stretch.

(Dorsiflexion of the feet may be added.)

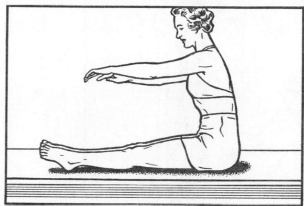

3. *Supine*, at end of table, hips flexed to 45 degrees, knees extended, heels resting against wall, arms partially abducted or hands behind neck.
a. Flex each hip through as complete a range as possible to stretch hamstrings. Hold and return slowly to position.
b. Move hips closer to wall as range increases (illustrated).

(Dorsiflexion of the foot may be added.)

A pad or small folded towel can be placed under the lumbar area of the spine to prevent too much tension in the lumbar extensors. The pelvis should be kept firmly against table.

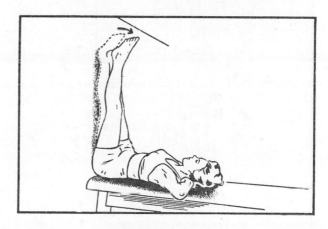

4. *Half sitting*, one leg on table, other partially supporting body weight.

Flex hip and use manual pressure (just above the knee) to extend the knee. The stretch may be increased by further hip flexion, if knee can be completely extended.

(Be sure heel can slide easily on table surface.)

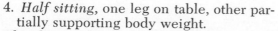

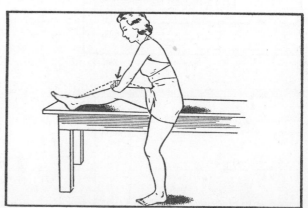

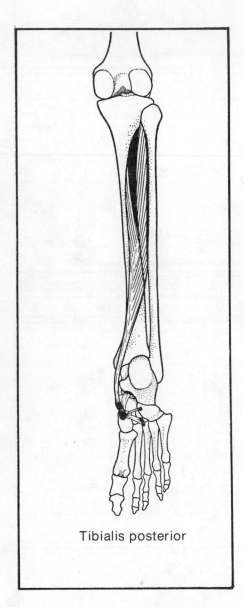

Tibialis posterior

FOOT INVERTOR

Tibialis Posterior

Origin: Proximal two thirds of medial surface of fibula, posterior tibia, and interosseous membrane.

Insertion: Tuberosity of navicular, with fibrous expansions to sustentaculum tali of the calcaneus, three cuneiforms, cuboid, and bases of second, third, and fourth metatarsal bones.

The tibialis posterior muscle is in an excellent position to support the long arch of the foot. It pulls upward and slightly backward from the apex of the arch (tuberosity on the medial side of the navicular bone). Its pull is extended over the plantar area of the foot through numerous fibrous expansions.

ALIGNMENT OF THE LOWER EXTREMITY

EXERCISES FOR LOCALIZING AND STRENGTHENING THE TIBIALIS POSTERIOR

1. *Sitting,* one ankle resting on opposite knee.
a. Plantar flex the ankle and invert the foot. Relax slowly.
(Have subject identify the tendon of the tibialis posterior and note the line of pull.)
b. Resist the motion by placing heel of hand against forefoot or resist in the same manner upon completion of motion. Relax slowly.

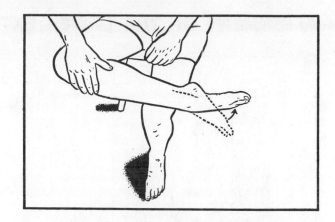

2. *Sitting,* feet parallel and slightly apart, legs vertical.
Raise the longitudinal arches, emphasizing the pull of the tibialis posterior muscles. Keep the knees in place and the heads of the metatarsal bones in firm contact with the floor.
(Attempting to shorten the foot without permitting the heel or any of the metatarsal heads or toes to leave the floor assists in localizing the motion.)

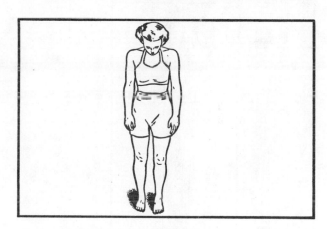

3. *Standing,* feet parallel, patellae in line with ankles.
Raise the arches, emphasizing the pull of the tibialis posterior muscles. The knees should be relaxed (not hyperextended) and the body weight evenly distributed over the feet. The heads of all the metatarsals of each foot should rest firmly on the floor.

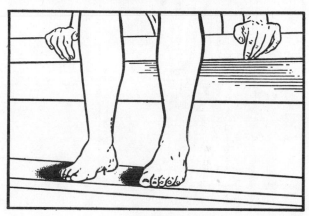

4. *Walking*
Attempt to maintain the long arch during the weight-bearing period of the step, and the patellae in line with the ankles.
Emphasize the pull of the tibialis posterior.

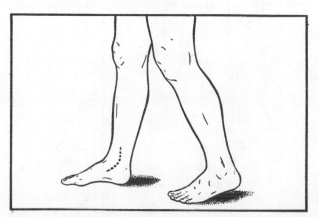

ALIGNMENT OF THE LOWER EXTREMITY

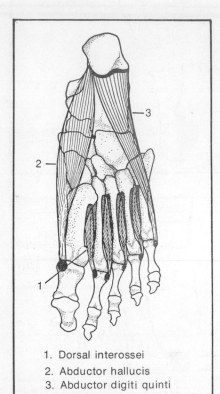

1. Dorsal interossei
2. Abductor hallucis
3. Abductor digiti quinti

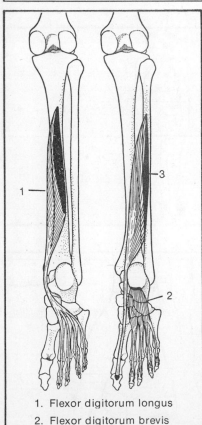

1. Flexor digitorum longus
2. Flexor digitorum brevis
3. Flexor hallucis longus

MUSCLES TO BE STRENGTHENED

ABDUCTORS OF THE TOES

Dorsal Interossei

Origin: Adjacent sides of the metatarsal bones.
Insertion: Base of proximal phalanges of second, third, and fourth toes.

Abductor Hallucis

Origin: Tuberosity of calcaneus.
Insertion: Medial side of first phalanx of hallux.

Abductor Digiti Quinti

Origin: Tuberosity and inferior surface of calcaneus.
Insertion: Lateral side of first phalanx of fifth toe.
In addition to the abductor action, the abductor hallucis and the abductor digiti quinti provide strong muscle struts which help to maintain the long arches of the foot.

FLEXORS OF THE TOES

Flexor Digitorum Longus

Origin: Posterior tibia.
Insertion: Bases of distal phalanges of lateral four toes.

Flexor Digitorum Brevis

Origin: Medial aspect of calcaneal tuberosity.
Insertion: Sides of second phalanges of lateral four toes.

Flexor Hallucis Longus

Origin: Posterior surface of fibula.
Insertion: Base of distal phalanx of hallux.
The flexor hallucis longus passes beneath the sustentaculum tali just medial to the weight-bearing portion of the calcaneus and its support aids in preventing calcaneal eversion.

Flexor Hallucis Brevis

(See page 94.)

ALIGNMENT OF THE LOWER EXTREMITY

EXERCISES FOR TOE ABDUCTORS

1. *Long sitting*
Abduct the toes.
(Abduction of toes in the beginning may be
   very difficult, especially of the hallux, because of disuse due to the constriction of
   shoes. Utilization of the intrinsic muscles
   of the foot helps to increase flexibility in
   the metatarsal area.)

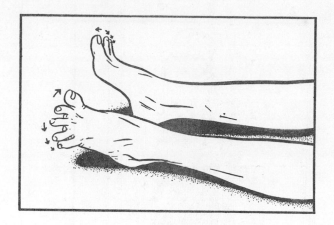

2. *Sitting*, feet resting on floor.
Abduct toes, attempting to avoid either
   flexion or extension at the metatarsophalangeal joints.
(Partial weight bearing is useful in the control of flexion and extension of toes during this exercise.)

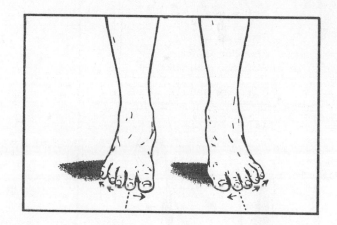

EXERCISE FOR TOE FLEXORS (LONG FLEXORS)

1. *Sitting*, legs slightly medially rotated,
   feet apart and resting on a bar or stool
   supporting the metatarsal heads but permitting free movement of toes.
Flex toes over edge (curl).
(Contraindicated if hammer toes present.
   See discussion page 94.)

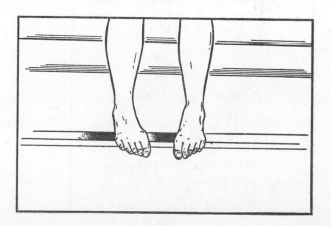

ALIGNMENT OF THE LOWER EXTREMITY

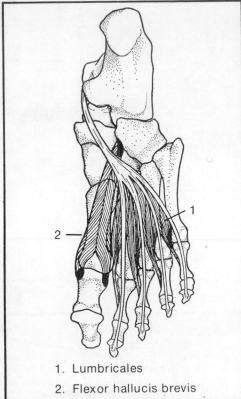

1. Lumbricales
2. Flexor hallucis brevis

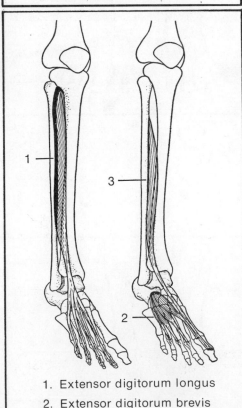

1. Extensor digitorum longus
2. Extensor digitorum brevis
3. Extensor hallucis longus

FLEXORS OF THE METATARSOPHALANGEAL JOINTS

Lumbricales

Origin: Tendons of flexor digitorum longus.

Insertion: Pass around toes to insert into tendons of extensor digitorum longus.

Flexor Hallucis Brevis

Origin: Cuboid and lateral cuneiform.

Insertion: Medial and lateral sides of base of proximal phalanx of hallux.

The lumbricales, flexor hallucis brevis, and the dorsal and plantar interossei (not illustrated) all flex the first metatarsophalangeal joints of the toes. The lumbricales, through their insertion into the flexor digitorum longus tendons, extend the middle and terminal phalanges of the four lateral toes. Flexion of the metatarsophalangeal joints with extension of the toes helps to correct hammer toes (hyperextension of the proximal phalanx together with flexion of the middle and distal phalanges). In hammer toes of long duration, both the flexor and extensor muscles may require stretching.

MUSCLES TO BE STRETCHED

EXTENSORS OF THE TOES

Extensor Digitorum Longus

Origin: Proximal three fourths of anterior surface of fibula.

Insertion: Second and third phalanges of lateral four toes.

Extensor Digitorum Brevis

Origin: Upper and lateral surfaces of calcaneus.

Insertion: Medial division into dorsal surface of base of proximal phalanx of hallux. Lateral three divisions into tendons of long extensors of second, third, and fourth toes.

Extensor Hallucis Longus

Origin: Anterior surface of fibula.

Insertion: Base of distal phalanx of hallux.

ALIGNMENT OF THE LOWER EXTREMITY

EXERCISES FOR STRENGTHENING TOE FLEXORS (LUMBRICALES) AND STRETCHING EXTENSORS OF INTERPHALANGEAL JOINTS OF THE TOES

1. *Sitting,* with heads of metatarsal bones supported by a bar or stool.

Flex toes at metatarsophalangeal joint, keeping distal joints straight.

(Range of motion may be increased by shifting knees forward and dorsiflexing the ankles, which decreases tension in the long toe extensors.)

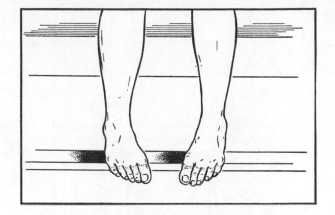

2. *Long sitting*

Flex the metatarsophalangeal joints of the toes, keeping the distal joints straight.

(Shortened long toe extensors may be stretched by partial, then complete, plantar flexion of ankles.)

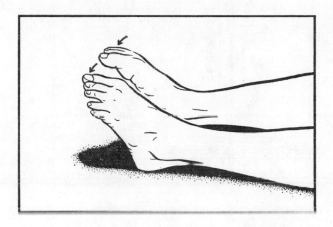

ALIGNMENT OF THE LOWER EXTREMITY

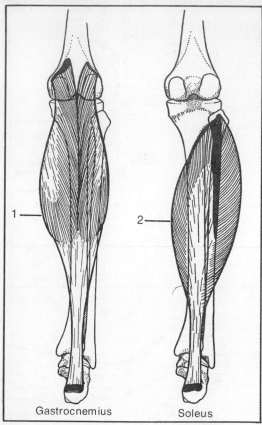

1 —

2 —

Gastrocnemius   Soleus

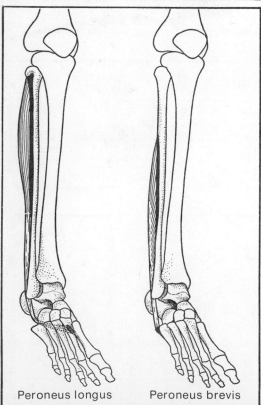

Peroneus longus   Peroneus brevis

ANKLE PLANTAR FLEXORS

Gastrocnemius

Origin: Medial and lateral heads from medial and lateral condyles of femur.

Insertion: Tendo calcaneus, inserting into posterior surface of calcaneus.

Soleus

Origin: Head and proximal third of fibular shaft, popliteal line, and middle third of tibia.

Insertion: Tendo calcaneus.

Because of the large cross-sectional area and favorable leverage of the calf muscles at the ankle, they can produce tremendous force with little danger of injury. Hence, they are utilized advantageously for pushing or lifting.

FOOT EVERTORS

Peroneus Longus

Origin: Head and proximal two thirds of lateral surface of fibula; occasional fibers from tibial condyle.

Insertion: Tendon passes behind lateral malleolus, forward to groove on cuboid, and beneath foot to lateral side of first metatarsal base and medial cuneiform.

Peroneus Brevis

Origin: Distal two thirds of lateral surface of body of fibula.

Insertion: Behind lateral malleolus to tuberosity of base of fifth metatarsal on lateral side of bone.

The peroneus longus is an important muscle in maintaining the arched position of the metatarsals (page 98).

ALIGNMENT OF THE LOWER EXTREMITY

EXERCISES FOR STRETCHING ANKLE PLANTAR FLEXORS

1. *Long sitting,* feet slightly apart and parallel.
Strongly plantar flex feet, avoiding inversion or eversion for gastrocnemius and soleus stretch.

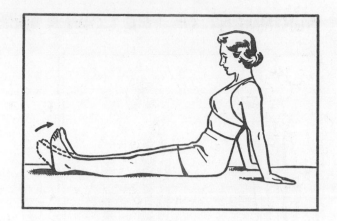

2. *Standing,* chair or table for support, feet parallel with slight inversion. One leg 12 to 19 inches in front of the other.
Shift body weight forward as far as possible, flexing knee, keeping the other leg extended. Both heels are kept in contact with floor.
Repeat, alternating legs.
(Knee flexion of the leg in front limits the stretch to the soleus as the gastrocnemius is slack. Knee extension of the back leg provides a combined gastrocnemius–soleus stretch. Keeping the feet parallel with slight inversion protects the arch. An in-toe position should be used if there is a tendency toward pronation.)

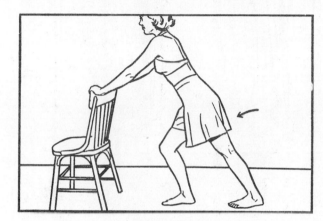

3. *Standing,* feet 12 to 18 inches from wall (see position of feet above), knees, hips, and spine extended.
Shift body weight forward from ankles as far as possible.

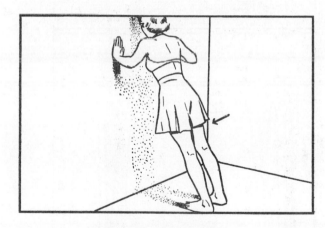

EXERCISE FOR STRETCHING FOOT EVERTORS

1. *Sitting,* one leg crossed over opposite knee.
Invert and adduct the foot, and dorsiflex the ankle, to stretch the peroneals. This is the action of the tibialis anterior (page 98).
If the tibialis anterior is hypertrophied, use manual pressure only for stretching (see discussion page 98). (Illustrated.)

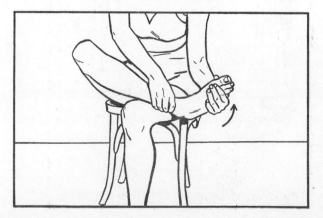

ALIGNMENT OF THE LOWER EXTREMITY

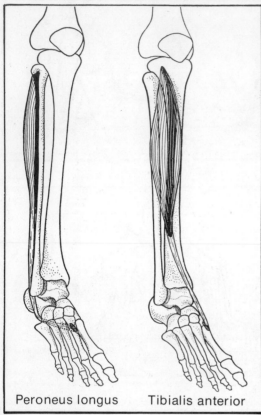

Peroneus longus   Tibialis anterior

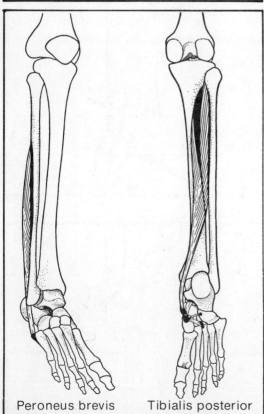

Peroneus brevis   Tibialis posterior

MUSCLES CONTROLLING LATERAL STABILITY OF THE FOOT

EVERTORS AND INVERTORS OF THE FOOT

Peroneus Longus

Origin and insertion (see page 96).

Tibialis Anterior

Origin: Lateral condyle and proximal two thirds of anterolateral surface of tibial body and interosseus membrane.

Insertion: Medial and plantar surfaces of first cuneiform bone and base of first metatarsal bone.

The peroneus longus, as has been pointed out (page 96) is an important factor in supporting the arched position of the metatarsal dome (page 79). Together with the tibialis anterior, which attaches medially on the same bones, it forms a sling or stirrup under the foot. The peroneus longus also is in a position to depress the first metatarsal segment in walking.

The tibialis anterior inserts so far forward on the medial side of the foot, that it is not in an advantageous position to maintain the longitudinal arch. When hypertrophied it may actually depress the arch.

Peroneus Brevis.

Origin and insertion (see page 96).

Tibialis Posterior

Origin and insertion (see page 90).

The peroneus brevis and the tibialis posterior are so placed that they help provide lateral stability for the foot. The tibialis posterior also supports the longitudinal arch (see page 90).

ALIGNMENT OF THE LOWER EXTREMITY

EXERCISES FOR LATERAL STABILITY OF THE FOOT (INVERTORS AND EVERTORS)

1. *Long sitting*
Dorsiflex one foot while plantar flexing the other. Pedal slowly, avoiding inversion or eversion.

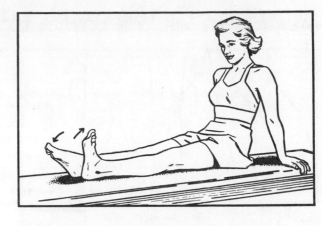

2. *Sitting* on chair in front of mirror
Raise one heel from floor and lower it as other heel is raised (pedaling). The ball of the foot and the toes should remain in contact with the floor. Avoid inversion or eversion of the foot.

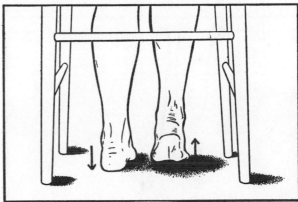

3. *Standing*, facing mirror
Raise the heel of one foot, gripping with the toes. As the heel is lowered, shift the body weight over that side while raising the opposite heel. Shift back and forth, elevating the body as high as possible without lateral or medial deviation of the feet.
Progression. Increase speed while maintaining balanced position of feet.

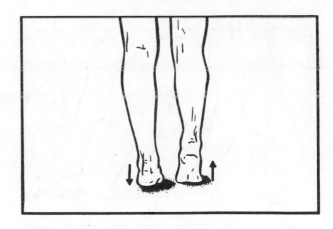

4. *Standing*
Walk slowly, avoiding inversion or eversion, gripping floor with toes on each step.
Progression. Increase speed while maintaining foot alignment.

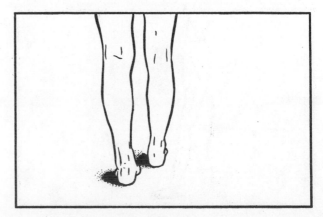

ALIGNMENT OF THE LOWER EXTREMITY

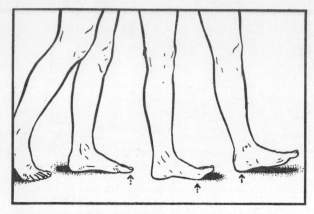

LOCALIZATION OF WEIGHT-BEARING AREAS

1. *Walking* (heel, ball, toes)
Place the heel, ball of foot, and toes down on the floor as three distinct and separate areas. Press downward with the toes and control lateral muscle balance during the supporting phase.

There should be slight lateral rotation at the hip, depending upon the alignment of the extremity.

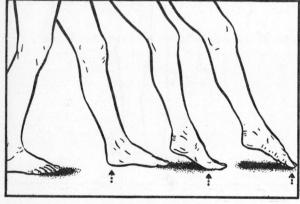

2. *Walking* (heel, ball, each toe)
Place heel on the floor, then the ball of the foot; then bring the toes to the floor one at a time, starting with the fifth toe and ending with the first.

Control of the intrinsic musculature of the foot is emphasized and attention is focused on the specific weight-bearing areas of the foot.

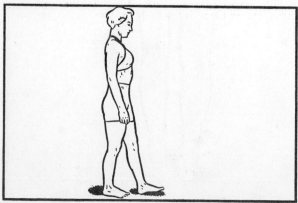

3. *Walking* (toes, ball, heel), slight lateral rotation at the hips.
Place the toes, then the ball of the foot, and finally the heel on the floor as three separate areas. All the toes touch the floor at the same time and grip the floor as the rest of the foot is lowered. The entire metatarsal area should be placed evenly on the floor.

The sequence of floor contact is reversed to gain flexibility and control of the position of the foot.

4. *Walking*
Keep in mind:
a) maintenance of the long arch of the foot during stance;
b) gripping action of the toes, pressing downward and aiding in balance and support in weight bearing;
c) conscious localization of weight-bearing areas; and
d) even balance of evertor and invertor muscle groups.
Progression. The speed of walking may be increased as proficiency improves.

IV DAILY ACTIVITIES AND REST

The entire purpose of the segmental exercises discussed in previous sections will be lost unless the individual becomes aware of static and dynamic positions of the body throughout the day. Fundamentals of good body mechanics can be adapted to the needs of each individual, but ingenuity is required of the instructor working with persons of various ages, interests, and occupations.

MECHANICS OF LIFTING

When the dynamics involved are analyzed, it is easy to understand why the low back region is subject to injury. Most daily activities require activity of the arms in front of the body, as in reaching and lifting, with accompanying forward inclination of the trunk. The farther the trunk is flexed forward, the more subject to strain are the supporting structures. The reasons are as follows: First, as the trunk flexes, the rotational movement resulting from gravitational pull is increased; this puts a greater load on the back extensor muscles and ligaments. Second, the angle of pull of the back muscles becomes less favorable with trunk flexion. This decrease in the effective component of these muscles in supporting the trunk necessitates an increase in muscle contraction force.

As a result of the decrease in the angle of pull and the increase in muscle force required, the compression force acting downward along the spinal column becomes tremendous (Fig. 19).

Strait and others estimate that the tensile force in the erector spinae muscles (page 25) necessary to support the trunk of a 180-pound man standing with his trunk flexed to 60 degrees from the vertical (with his arms hanging freely) must be approximately 450 pounds. If he holds a 50-pound weight, the muscle force must be *750 pounds,* and the resultant compression

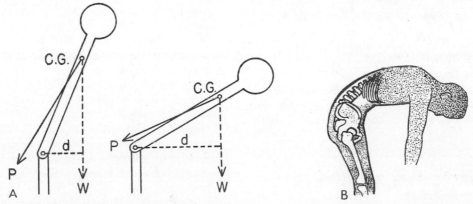

Figure 19.   Idealized illustration of trunk flexion to approximately 60 degrees. The combined weight of the head, arms and trunk (W) acts at the center of gravity (C.G.). The base of the spine, or lumbosacral joint, is shown as a fixed fulcrum. P represents the effective muscle tension exerted by the spinal extensors. The torque exerted by gravity, W × d, is greatly increased in position B, putting a tremendous load on the low back structures, particularly if a weight is carried in the hands. (Adapted from Strait, et al., by permission of the authors.)

force on the fifth lumbar vertebra is nearly *850 pounds.* It is not surprising, therefore, that low back injuries are common and that the fifth lumbar intervertebral disk is the one most frequently ruptured.

The stress placed on the low back structures as a result of even a slight forward inclination of the trunk is apparent to the individual suffering from acute low back pain. For him, such mild activities as leaning forward to brush his teeth or put on his shoes become major problems. Even before he is told to keep his trunk in a vertical position, such a person will carefully do so in order to avoid further pain. This guarded trunk position is the basic consideration guiding activity posture.

Motions should be smooth and steady when force is exerted in lifting, with muscles properly "set" in preparation for handling the weight (ready to respond if weight is heavier than anticipated).

PREVENTION OF STRAIN AND EARLY FATIGUE

Every effort should be made to avoid strain and early fatigue in work or recreation. Attention to body position and activity environment are therefore essential.

POSITIONS FOR ACTIVITIES

1. The trunk should be kept as erect as possible.
2. Slight hyperextension of the lumbar spine, as in the normal standing position, should be retained when work is done in front or to the side of the body. Conversely, care should be taken in lifting heavy objects over the head when hyperextension is increased in the lumbar area of the spine.
3. A wide stance, with one foot to the side or in front of the other, provides increased stability and allows a shift of the body weight with minimum inclination of the trunk.
4. Loads should be carried close to the body in order to bring the weight as near as possible to the vertical gravity line.
5. Knees should be *only* partially flexed when lifting objects from the floor. Below an angle of approximately 65 degrees, the efficiency of the quadriceps muscles begins to decrease sharply and the strain on the knee joints is greatly increased.

ADJUSTING THE ACTIVITY ENVIRONMENT

There are a number of ways in which the activity environment can be accommodated to the individual. Among them are the adjustment of working surfaces, the design of equipment, the arrangement of materials, and the selection of chairs.

Adjustment of Working Surfaces

Surfaces of tables, counters, etc., should be at a height which permits working with the trunk erect.

Equipment Design

Equipment should be designed for ample leg space during sitting and toe space when standing.

Arrangement of Materials

Any materials that are required should be so placed that strain is not entailed in obtaining or placing them. Heavy objects should not be on or near the floor or far above the level of the working surface.

Selection of Chairs

Care should be taken in selecting chairs to be used for prolonged periods of work in office or home, when the body must be maintained in an erect position, and in selecting those for relaxed reading or rest. It appears impractical and usually is unrewarding to admonish individuals to maintain good alignment when chairs are ill-fitting and offer little support for long-time sitting. Ideally, work chairs should be adjustable, to offer the best possible fit for all persons who use them (page 107). At least, when one is purchased for an individual, the elements needed should receive consideration. The objectives are to provide stability of body structures for good alignment and to permit muscle relaxation for comfort.

Blanton presents an interesting description of the interaction between a sitter and a chair with a seat depth that was too great. According to his observations of time-lapse films, a particular series of events occurred many times. In each case, the sitter slid into a backward slumped position, propped himself up first with his arms, crossed his knees and then stretched both legs forward, ending in a nearly horizontal position. In terms of interaction, the seat slowly and repeatedly ejected the sitter.

Akerblom and many other researchers have emphasized the need for support of the lumbar area of the spine and the proper height and size of the chair seat for erect sitting.

Grandjean and his collaborators have designed a profile of a chair that will offer support to the physiological curves of the body during periods of relaxed reading or rest (page 107). In addition, the researchers have presented a profile that offers further support to the sacral region of the back for individuals who have low back discomfort or pain.

INTERVALS OF REST

Intervals of rest before, during, and after exercise are indicated in the early treatment of persons who fatigue quickly. If the positions are used over extensive periods of time, exercises to maintain the length of the flexor muscles of the lower extremities should be carried out concurrently, as they tend to shorten when adjacent joints are supported in recumbency.

POSITIONS OF THE BODY IN ACTIVITY AND REST

Analysis of ordinary daily activities shows that motions consist of a few fundamental components which are variously combined. These are illustrated in the following pages and include stooping, lifting, carrying, reaching, and the application of body weight in activities such as pushing, pulling, or supporting.

Sitting alignment in prolonged work situations that require the erect position and in rest positions, including relaxed reading, are also included. Recommendations are made for the selection of chairs for both erect sitting and relaxed positions. Recumbent rest positions are described for use at home and during intervals of rest between exercises.

The physical therapist has three opportunities for the use of this information: 1) the teaching of patients suffering from the effects of injury; 2) the instructing of individuals in prevention of strain and injury; and 3) the practicing of good body mechanics in his own work, to eliminate as much strain and fatigue as possible.

POSITIONS OF THE BODY IN ACTIVITY

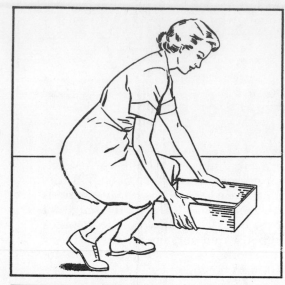

STOOPING AND LIFTING

Correct Method

The trunk should be as erect as possible, with knees partially flexed.

The load is held close to body to keep all weight near the center of gravity.

The feet are well apart, with one foot forward for a stable base of support.

The plantar flexors of the feet are used as much as possible because of their strength.

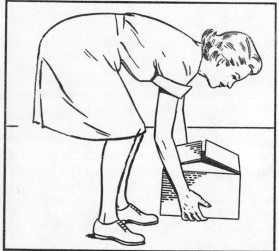

Incorrect Method

The back is in full flexion, with trunk far forward, placing a great strain on the lumbar area.

The feet are close together and almost parallel, offering a limited base of support (see Fig. 19, page 101).

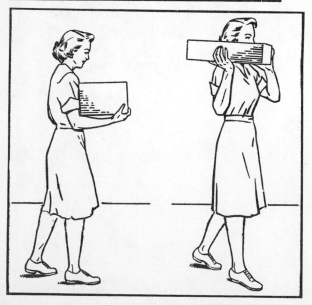

CARRYING

Correct Methods

In the illustration on the left, the load is supported near the body to minimize the strain on the back.

On the right, the load is carried on the shoulder or at shoulder level (waitress position) to bring the center of the weight nearer to the midline of the body.

POSITIONS OF THE BODY IN ACTIVITY

REACHING WITH PUSHING OR PULLING

Correct Method

Arms and shoulders are fixed against the thorax in massage, and the whole body moves forward from the ankles with knee flexion.

A wide stance, with the forward foot directed in the line of movement, allows the effective use of the body weight in exerting pressure and the minimum use of the back extensors for return to position.

Incorrect Method

Arms, shoulders, and upper trunk only are used to exert pressure.

The narrow stance prohibits a forward movement of the pelvis and lower extremities and requires intensive use of the back extensor muscles leading to unnecessary strain and fatigue.

Correct Method (Left Figure Below)

The feet are separated in a wide stance, in activities such as making a bed or plinth.

Forward movement primarily at the ankle joints allows the trunk to maintain a more vertical position.

Incorrect Method (Right Figure Below)

A narrower stance with knees remaining in extension brings about unnecessary hip flexion with strain on the back extensor muscles.

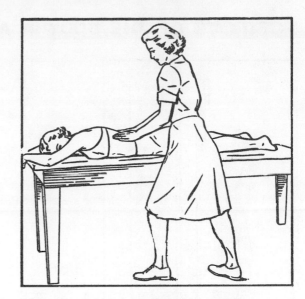

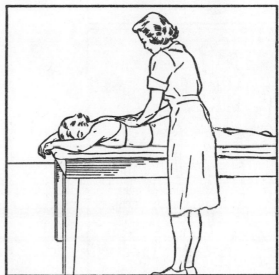

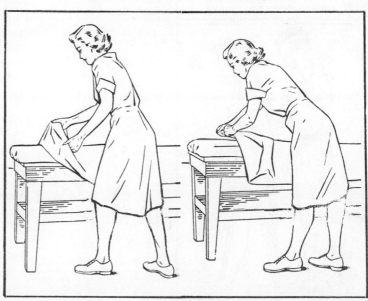

POSITIONS OF THE BODY IN ACTIVITY

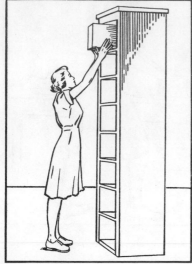

REACHING AND LIFTING

A heavy load should not be placed on the lumbar spine when it is in a position of increased hyperextension. If equipment is stored on a high shelf, a stool would help to eliminate this hazard.

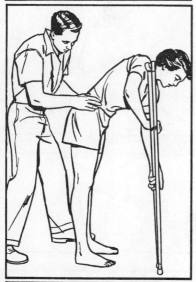

ASSISTING WITH CRUTCH WALKING

Positioning for effective use of the body is necessary in assisting or guarding a patient who is learning functional activities. For example, in crutch walking, the therapist must constantly adjust his position and be ready to instantly exert the necessary force to steady the patient or to catch him if he falls.

In preparation for crutch walking, the therapist stands close to the patient, with a wide stance and one foot well forward for stability.

Light contact of the hands on the pelvis makes it possible to provide support, if needed, or to give the patient a sense of security. It also allows him to instantly detect off-balance movements or a tendency for the knees to flex, leading to a fall.

In the swing-through gait, the therapist's step must be closely coordinated with the movements of the patient to prevent a fall. Light hand pressure on one shoulder and on the opposite side of the pelvis allows control of the patient's trunk.

Keeping one foot well forward on each step, the therapist can bring the patient's weight back against his thigh if the patient begins to fall.

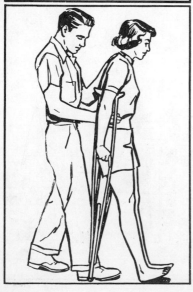

POSITIONS OF THE BODY IN ACTIVITY AND REST

SITTING ALIGNMENT

WORKING

In the illustration on the left, the figure has good alignment; however, this position can only be maintained for a very short period of time in the chair depicted. Slumping (illustration on the right) soon occurs, with strain on the lumbar spine and undue flexion of the thoracic and cervical areas.

The chair in the illustration on the left should have a lower seat to relieve pressure under the thighs from the front edge. The horizontal panel across the back should be lower to support the concavity of the lumbar spine, which will aid in maintaining the vertical balance of the upper spine and head. The contours of the pelvis and hips should fit well back in the open space for a solid base and good balance.

Some form of upholstery for the seat and back is important in relieving the pressures caused by long-term work periods.

The posture chair (illustrated) can provide the support needed through adjustment of the seat and back. If purchase of such a chair is not practical, the basic elements should be considered in selecting a work chair for any individual.

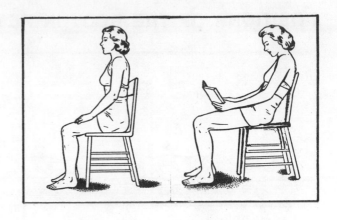

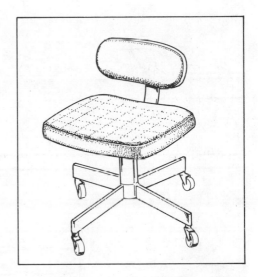

RELAXED READING OR RESTING

The seat profile illustrated was developed through experimentation for reading or rest.* Note the support given to the physiological curves. The designers recommend:

Reading—seat inclination   23–24°
            back-rest inclination   101–104°
Rest   —seat inclination   25– 26°
            back-rest inclination   105–108°
Upholstery (dark area)—6 cm. thick

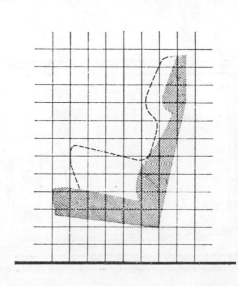

*Illustration from Grandjean, E., et al.: Ergonomics, *12*:307–315, 1969.

POSITIONS OF THE BODY IN REST

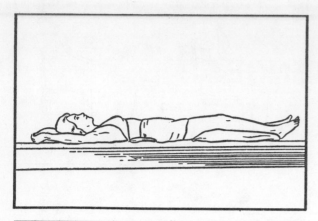

Backlying (Supine)

Place appropriate size pillows under head and knees, pad or folded towel under lumbar area of the spine.

Place arms in the most comfortable position for the person. Arms are abducted in the illustration to show pad under the lumbar area.

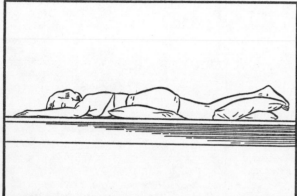

Facelying (Prone)

Place a pillow under the hips, a second pillow under the ankles. The arms should be in a comfortable position and the head turned to one side.

If there is flexibility in the shoulders, the reverse T position for the arms may aid relaxation by relieving the downward drag of the shoulder girdle (illustrated).

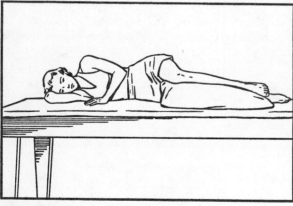

Sidelying

The upper leg is flexed and supported by one or more pillows, according to the width of the pelvis, to avoid twisting of body segments. The head also should be elevated to remain in line with the spine.

The upper arm is placed in position to support the trunk (illustrated). Further relaxation can be obtained by placing a pillow against the trunk, supporting the upper arm, so that the trunk will not roll forward.

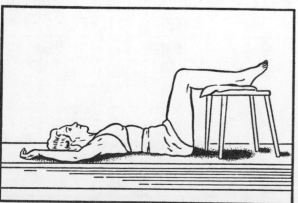

Backlying (Supine) with hips and knees flexed at right angles, supported by padded stool or pillows.

Place arms in reverse T (as illustrated) or at sides.

REFERENCES

Akerblom, V. B. Anatomische und Physiologische Grundlagen zur Gestaltung von Sitzen. Ergonomics, 12:120–131, 1969.

Allsop, K. G. Potential Hazards of Abdominal Exercises. J. Health, P. E. and Rec., 42:1:89, 1971.

Bak, E. I. Exercise Therapy of Posturally Defective School Children. Phys. Ther. Rev., 37:287–291, 1957.

Barlow, W. Anxiety and Muscle-Tension Pain. Brit. J. Clin. Pract., 13:339–350, 1959.

Barlow, W. Posture and Its Re-education, Therapeutic Exercise, Edited by S. Licht, New Haven, E. Licht, Publisher, 1961.

Barlow, W. Psychosomatic Problems in Postural Re-education. Lancet, 2:659–664, 1955.

Barnett, C. H. Locking at the Knee Joint. J. Anat., 87:91–95, 1953.

Bartholomew, D. R., and Vernon, W. G. Rapid Rehabilitation of the Injured Back in an Industrial Environment. Phys. Ther. Rev., 40:875–877, 1960.

Basmajian, J. V. Man's Posture. Arch. Phys. Med., 46:26–36, 1965.

Basmajian, J. V. Muscles Alive: Their Functions Revealed by Electromyography. 3rd ed. Baltimore, Williams and Wilkins Company, 1974.

Borelli, J. A. De Motu Animalium. Rome, 1680.

Bradford, D. S., Moe, J. H., and Winter, R. B. Kyphosis and Postural Round Back Deformity in Children and Adolescents. Minn. Med., 56:114–120, 1973.

Branton, P. Behavior, Body Mechanics and Discomfort. Ergonomics, 12:316–327, 1969.

Braune, C. W., and Fischer, O. Uber die Lage des Schwerpunktes des menschlichen Körpers, Col. XV: Abh. Math. Phys. Klasse d. Kgl. Sachsen, Ges. d. Wiss. Leipzig, S. Hirzel, 1889.

Brennan, J. F. A Comparative Analysis of Upright Posture as the Foundation of Individual Psychology. J. Individ. Psych., 24:25–32, 1968.

Brunnstrom, S. Center of Gravity Line in Relation to Ankle Joint in Erect Standing: Application to Posture Training and to Artificial Legs. Phys. Ther. Rev., 34:109–115, 1954.

Cailliet, R. Neck and Arm Pain. Philadelphia, F. A. Davis Company, 1964.

Cailliet, R. Low Back Pain Syndrome. Philadelphia, F. A. Davis Company, 1968.

Campbell, E. J. M., Agostoni, E., and Davis, J. N. The Respiratory Muscles: Mechanics and Neural Control. Philadelphia, W. B. Saunders Company, 1970.

Carlsoo, S. Influence of Frontal and Dorsal Loads on Muscle Activity and on the Weight Distribution in the Feet. Acta Orthop. Scandinav., 34:299–309, 1964.

Christaldi, J., and Mueller, G. W. Let's Do Something about Posture Education. J. Health, P. E. and Rec., 34:1:14, and 34:2:28, 1963.

Clarke, H. H. An Objective Method of Measuring the Height of the Longitudinal Arch of the Foot. Research Quart., 3:99, 1933.

Clarke, H. H. The Application of Measurement to Health and Physical Education. New York, Prentice-Hall, 1945.

Clarke, H. H., and Clarke, D. H. Developmental and Adaptive Physical Education. New York, Prentice-Hall, 1963.

Cureton, T. K. The Validity of Antero-Posterior Spinal Measurements. Research Quart., 2:101–113, 1931.

Cureton, T. K. Physical Fitness Appraisal and Guidance. St. Louis, The C. V. Mosby Company, 1947.

Cureton, T. K. The Physiological Effects of Exercise Programs on Adults. Springfield, Illinois, Charles C Thomas, 1971.

Daniels, L., and Worthingham, C. Muscle Testing, Techniques of Manual Examination. 3rd ed. Philadelphia, W. B. Saunders Company, 1972.

Doane, K. R. Differences Between Pupils With Good Sitting Posture and Pupils With Poor Sitting Posture. J. Ed. Res., 52:315–317, 1959.

duBois-Reymond, R. Handbuch der Physiologie des Menschen. Vol. IV, Nagel Braunschweig, 1905.

Egli, H. Bases for Selection of Mobilization Techniques. Phys. Ther. Rev., 38:759–761, 1958.

Eldred, E. Posture and Locomotion. Handbook of Physiology, Sect. 1, Neurophysiology. Washington, D. C., Am. Physiological Society, 1959.

Elftman, H. A Cinematic Study of the Distribution of Pressure in the Human Foot. Anat. Rec., 59:481–491, 1934.

Ellfeldt, L., and Lowman, C. L. Exercises for the Mature Adult. Springfield, Illinois, Charles C Thomas, 1973.

Falkner, F. T., (ed.). Human Development. Philadelphia, W. B. Saunders Company, 1966.

Fick, R. Handbuch der Anatomie und Mechanik der Gelenke. Jena, G. Fischer, 1911.

Flint, M. M. An Electromyographic Comparison of the Functions of the Iliacus and the Rectus Abdominis Muscles: a Preliminary Report. J. Amer. Phys. Ther. Assoc., 45:248–253, 1965.

Flint, M. M., and Diehl, B. Influence of Abdominal Strength, Back Extensor Strength and Trunk Strength Balance Upon Antero-posterior Alignment of Elementary School Girls. Research Quart. 32:490–498, 1961.

Floyd, W. F., and Silver, P. H. S. Electromyographic Study of Standing in Man: Thigh and Leg Muscles. J. Physiol., 111:22–26, 1950.

Floyd, W. F., and Ward, J. S. Anthropometric and Physiological Considerations in School, Office and Factory Seating. Ergonomics, 12:132–139, 1969.

Ford, A. B. Energy Cost of Work. Phys. Ther. Rev., 40:859–862, 1960.

Fox, M. G., and Young, O. G. Placement of the Gravital

Line in Anteroposterior Standing Posture. Research Quart., 25:277–285, 1954.

Gardiner, M. D. The Principles of Exercise Therapy. London, G. Bell and Sons, Ltd., 1957.

Gardner, E., Gray, D. J., and O'Rahilly, R. Anatomy—A Regional Study of Human Structure. 4th ed. Philadelphia, W. B. Saunders Company, 1975.

Gaskell, D. V., and Webber, B. A. The Brompton Hospital Guide to Chest Physiotherapy. 2nd ed. Oxford, Blackwell Scientific Publications, 1973.

Goldthwaite, J. E., Brown, L. T., Swain, L. T., and Kuhn, J. G. Essentials of Body Mechanics in Health and Disease. 5th ed. Philadelphia, J. B. Lippincott Company, 1952.

Grandjean, E., Boni, A., and Kretzschmar, H. The Development of a Rest Chair Profile for Healthy and Notalgic People. Ergonomics, 12:307–315, 1969.

Grant, J. C. B. A Method of Anatomy, Descriptive and Deductive. 5th ed. Baltimore, Williams & Wilkins Company, 1952.

Grant, J. C. B. A Method of Anatomy; by Regions, Descriptive and Deductive. 9th ed. Edited by Basmajian, J. V., Baltimore, Williams and Wilkins Company, 1975.

Gray, H. Anatomy of the Human Body. 28th ed. Edited by Goss, C. M., Philadelphia, Lea and Febiger, 1966.

Gray, H. Gray's Anatomy. 35th ed. British ed. Edited by Warwick, R., and Williams, P. L., Philadelphia, W. B. Saunders Company, 1973.

Guten, B., and Lipetz, S. Electromyographic Investigation of the Rectus Abdominis in Abdominal Exercises. Research Quart., 42:256–263, 1971.

Haller, J. S., and Gurewitsch, A. O. An Approach to Dynamic Posture Based on Primitive Motion Patterns. Arch. Phys. Med., 31:632–640, 1950.

Harless, E. Die statischen Momente der menschlichen Gliedmassen. Akad. d. Wissensch. zu München, Abhandl. d. mathem.-physik. Klasses d. Kgl. Bayer, 8, 1857.

Hellebrandt, F. A. Standing as a Geotropic Reflex: The Mechanism of the Asynchronous Rotation of Motor Units. Am. J. Physiol., 121:471–474, 1938.

Hellebrandt, F. A., and Franseen, E. B. Physiological Study of Vertical Stance of Man. Physiol. Rev., 23:220–225, 1943.

Hellebrandt, F. A., and Fries, E. C. The Constancy of Oscillograph Stance Patterns. Physiotherapy Rev., 22:17–22, 1942.

Hellebrandt, F. A., and Fries, E. C. The Eccentricity of the Mean Vertical Projection of the Center of Gravity During Standing. Physiotherapy Rev., 22:186–192, 1942.

Hislop, H. J. Pain and Exercise. Phys. Ther. Rev., 40:98–106, 1960.

Hislop, H. J. The Penalties of Physical Disability. Phys. Ther., 58:271–278, 1976.

Hoefer, P. F. A. Innervation and "Tonus" of Striated Muscle in Man. Arch. Neurol. & Psychiat., 46:947–972, 1941.

Homola, S. Increase Lung Capacity With Chest-Expanding Exercise. Schol. Coach, 35:6:24, 1966.

Homola, S. Posture and Body Mechanics. Schol. Coach, 36:6:66, 1967.

Homola, S. Effects of Toe-Touching and Sit-Up Exercises Upon the Spine. Schol. Coach, 38:1:40, 1969.

Hunsacker, P. A., and Gray, G. Studies in Human Strength. Research Quart., 28:109–122, 1957.

Illingworth, R. S. The Development of the Infant and Young Child. 5th ed. Edinburgh, Churchill Livingstone, 1972.

Jacobson, E. You Must Relax. New York, McGraw-Hill Book Company, 1957.

Jacobson, E. Tension in Medicine. Springfield, Ill., Charles C Thomas, 1967.

Jones, H. H. Valsalva Procedure: Its Clinical Importance to the Physical Therapist. J. Amer. Phys. Ther. Assoc., 45:570–572, 1965.

Jones, J. C. Methods and Results of Seating Research. Ergonomics, 12:171–181, 1969.

Jones, L. The Postural Complex: Observations as to Cause, Diagnosis and Treatment. Springfield, Ill., Charles C Thomas, 1955.

Jones, R. L. The Human Foot—an Experimental Study of Its Mechanics and the Role of Its Muscles and Ligaments in the Support of the Arch. Am. J. Anat., 68:1–40, 1941.

Joseph, J. Man's Posture: Electromyographic Studies. Springfield, Ill., Charles C Thomas, 1960.

Joseph, J., and Nightingale, A. Electromyography of Muscles of Posture: Leg Muscles in Males. J. Physiol., 117:484–491, 1952.

Keith, A. Man's Posture: Its Evolution and Disorders. (Hunterian Lectures). Clin. Orthop., 62:5–14, 1969.

Kelton, I. W., and Wright, R. D. The Mechanism of Easy Standing in Man. Austral. J. Exper. Biol. & M. Sc., 27:505–515, 1949.

Kendall, F. P. A Criticism of Current Tests and Exercises for Physical Fitness. J. Amer. Phys. Ther. Assoc., 45:187–197, 1965.

Kendall, H. O., and Kendall, F. P. Developing and Maintaining Good Posture. J. Amer. Phys. Ther. Assoc., 48:319–336, 1968.

Kendall, H. O., Kendall, F. P., and Boynton, D. A. Posture and Pain. Baltimore, Williams & Wilkins, 1952.

Kent, B. E. Anatomy of the Trunk: A Review. Phys. Ther., Part I, 54:722–744, Part II, 54:850–860, 1974.

Knott, M., and Voss, D. E. Proprioceptive Neuromuscular Facilitation. New York, Harper and Row, 1968.

Kroemer, K. H. Seating in Plant and Office. Am. Ind. Hyg. Assoc. J., 32:633–652, 1971.

Kubicek, K., and Kubickova, B. The Prophylaxis of Faulty Posture. J. Sch. Health, 35:265–267, 1965.

Licht, S., and Johnson, E. W. Therapeutic Exercise. 2nd ed. New Haven, E. Licht, Publisher, 1961.

Lorusso, N. D. Physical Therapy for Low Back Pain. Phys. Ther. Rev., 40:878–880, 1960.

Lowman, C. L. Faulty Posture in Relation to Performance. J. Health, P. E., and Rec., 29:4:14, 1958.

Lowman, C. L., and Young, C. H. Posture and Fitness: Significance and Variances. Philadelphia, Lea and Febiger, 1960.

MacConaill, M. A., and Basmajian, J. V. Muscles and Movements; a Basis for Human Kinesiology. Baltimore, Williams & Wilkins Company, 1969.

McKenzie, J. The Foot as a Half-dome. Br. Med. J., 1:1068–1070, 1955.

Mathews, D. Measurement in Physical Education. Philadelphia, W. B. Saunders Company, 4th ed., 1973.

Mehrabian, A. Significance of Posture and Position in the Communication of Attitude and Status Relationships. Psychol. Bull., 71:359–372, 1969.

Mendler, H. M. Relationship of Hip Abductor Muscles to Posture. J. Amer. Phys. Ther. Assoc., 44:98–102, 1964.

Metheny, E. Body Dynamics. New York, McGraw-Hill Book Company, 1952.

Meyer, H. Das aufrechte Stehen. Arch. f. Anat., Phys. u. wissensch. Med., Jahrg., 9–45, 1853.

Meyer, H. Die wechselnde Lage des Schwerpunktes in menschlichen Körper. Leipzig, Engelmann, 1868.

Michele, A. A. Iliopsoas; Development of Anomalies in Man. Springfield, Ill., Charles C Thomas, 1962.

Miyazaki, A., and Sakou, T. Posture and Low Back Pain—Electromyographical Evaluation. Electromyography, 8:190–195, 1968.

Mommsen, G. Über die Sicherung des Kniegelenkes bei Amputationen und Lähmungen. Ztschr. f. Orth. Chir., 50:734–752, 1928.

Morton, D. J. The Human Foot; Its Evolution. Physiology and Functional Disorders. New York, Columbia University Press, 1935.

Morton, D. J., and Fuller, D. D. Human Locomotion and Body Form; a Study of Gravity and Man. Baltimore, Williams & Wilkins Company, 1952.

Mott, J. A. Conditioning and Basic Movement Concepts. Dubuque, William C. Brown Company, 1968.

Murray, M. P., Seireg, A., and Scholtz, R. C. Center of Gravity, Center of Pressure, and Supportive Forces During Human Activities. J. App. Physiol., 23:831–838, 1967.

Neuberger, T. Low Back Pain. Athletic J., 47:10:40, 1966.

Newton, K. Preventing Back Strain in Nursing. Am. J. Nursing, 43:921–924, 1943.

Palmer, C. E. Studies of the Center of Gravity in the Human Body. Child Develop., 15:99–180, 1944.

Partridge, M. J., and Walters, C. E. Participation of the Abdominal Muscles in Various Movements of the Trunk in Man. Phys. Ther. Rev., 39:791–800, 1959.

Peters, R. M. The Mechanical Basis of Respiration; an Approach to Respiratory Pathophysiology. Boston, Little, Brown Company, 1969.

Phillips, K. E. Evaluation of the Hip. Phys. Ther., 55:975–981, 1975.

Potts, P. Role of the Physical Therapist in Human Factors Engineering. Phys. Ther. Rev., 40:862–865, 1960.

Ralston, H. J. Some Considerations of the Physiological Bases of Therapeutic Exercise. Phys. Ther. Rev., 38:465–468, 1958.

Ralston, H. J., and Libet B. The Question of Tonus in Skeletal Muscle. Am. J. Phys. Med., 32:85–92, 1953.

Rathbone, J. L. Relaxation. Philadelphia, Lea and Febiger, 1969.

Rathbone, J. L., and Hunt, V. V. Corrective Physical Education. 7th ed. Philadelphia, W. B. Saunders Company, 1965.

Reeder, T. Electromyographic Study of the Latissimus Dorsi Muscle. J. Amer. Phys. Ther. Assoc., 43:165–172, 1963.

Reynolds, E. S., and Lovett, R. W. Method of Determining the Position of the Center of Gravity and Its Relation to Certain Bony Landmarks in Erect Position. Am. J. Physiol., 24:286–293, 1909.

Rogers, M. H. Basic Body Mechanics; an Interpretation. J. Health, P. E. and Rec., 32:12:20, 1961.

Roseborough, R. M., and Wilder, M. H. Postural Alignments as Applied to Problems in Reading. Acad. Therapy Q., 5:27–31, 1969.

Royal Committee for Working Conditions, Sweden. The Right Way to Lift and Carry. Phys. Ther. Rev., 38:99–103, 1958.

Ruch, T. C., and Patton, H. D. Physiology and Biophysics. Philadelphia, W. B. Saunders Company, 1974.

Scheidt, W. Untersuchungen über die Massenproportionen des menschlichen Körpers. Ztschr. f. Konstitutionslehre, 8:259–268, 1922.

Schwartz, R. P., and Heath, A. L. The Definition of Human Locomotion on the Basis of Measurement; with Description of Oscillographic Method. J. Bone Joint. Surg., 29:203–214, 1947.

Sheldon, W. H., Dupertuis, C. W., and McDermott, E. Atlas of Men. New York, Harper and Brothers, 1954.

Sheldon, W. H., Stevens, S. S., and Tucker, W. B. The Varieties of Human Physique. 4th ed. New York, Harper and Brothers, 1940.

Singleton, M., and LeVeau, B. F. The Hip Joint: Structure, Stability, and Stress. Phys. Ther., 55:957–968, 1975.

Smith, J. W. Observations on the Postural Mechanism of the Human Knee Joint. J. Anat., 90:236–261, 1956.

Smith, J. W. The Act of Standing. Acta Orthop. Scand., 23:159–168, 1953.

Smith, J. W. The Forces Operating at the Human Ankle Joint During Standing. J. Anat., 91:545–564, 1957.

Soderberg, G. L. Exercises for Abdominal Muscles. J. Health, P. E. and Rec., 37:9:67, 1966.

Steindler, A. Kinesiology of the Human Body. Springfield, Ill., Charles C Thomas, 1965.

Stevens, D. L., and Tomlinson, G. E. Measurement of Human Postural Sway. Proc. Roy. Soc. Med., 64:653–665, 1971.

Stone, R. E. Relationship between the Perception and Reproduction of Body Postures. Research Quart., 39:721–727, 1968.

Strait, L. A., Inman, V. T., and Ralston, H. J. Sample Illustrations of Physical Principles Selected from Physiology and Medicine. Am. J. Physics, 15:375–382, 1947.

Straus, E. W. Upright Posture. Psychiatric Quart., 26:529–561, 1952.

Tanigawa, M. C. Comparison of the Hold-relax Procedure and Passive Mobilization on Increasing Muscle Length. Phys. Ther., 52:725–735, 1972.

Tawast-Rancken, S. Posture Education in Finland. Phys. Ther. Rev., 37:298–301, 1957.

Thomas, D. P., and Whitney, L. Postural Movements During Normal Standing in Man. J. Anat., 93:524–539, 1959.

Treganza, A., and Fryman, V. M. Explorations into Posture and Body Mechanics. Acad. Therapy Q., 8:339–344, 1973.

Turner, M. Posture and Pain. Phys. Ther. Rev., 37:294–297, 1957.

Walsh, F. P., and Houtz, S. J. Attitudinal Deformities of the Lower Extremities in Small Children. Phys. Ther. Rev., 38:159–162, 1958.

Warren, C. G., Lehmann, J. F., and Koblanski, J. N. Heat and Stretch Procedures: An Evaluation Using Rat Tail Tendon. Arch. Phys. Med. Rehabil., 57:122–126, 1976.

Weber, W., and Weber, E. Mechanik der menschlichen Gehwerkzeuge. Göttingen, Dieterich, 1836.

Wells, K. F. What We Don't Know About Posture. J. Health, P. E. and Rec., 29:5–31, 1958.

Wells, K. F. Posture Exercise Handbook: A Progressive Sequence Approach. New York, The Ronald Press Company, 1963.

Wells, K. F. Kinesiology; the Scientific Base of Human Motion. Philadelphia, W. B. Saunders Company, 1971.

Williams, M., and Lissner, H. Biomechanics of Human Motion. Philadelphia, W. B. Saunders Company, 1962.

Williams, M., and Lissner, H. R. Biomechanical Analysis of Knee Function. J. Amer. Phys. Ther. Assoc., 43:93–99, 1963.

Williams, M., and Stutzman, L. Strength Variation Through the Range of Joint Motion. Phys. Ther. Rev., 39:145–152, 1959.

Worthingham, C. Study of Basic Physical Therapy Education: V. Request (Prescription or Referral) for Physical Therapy. J. Amer. Phys. Ther. Assoc., 50:989–1031, 1970.

INDEX

Note: In this Index, page numbers
in *italic* type refer to illustrations.

Habit, and posture, 1
Hallux valgus, 21, *21*
Hammer toes, 21, *21*
  exercise for correction of, 80, 84
Hamstrings, 31, *31*, 51, *51*, 88, *88*
  exercises for stretching, 87, *87*, 89, *89*
  test for limited motion, 31, *31*
Harrison's groove, 19, *19*
Head, forward inclination of, 12, *12*
Head tilt, 15, *15*
Hip, abductor muscles of, 28, *28*, 82, *82*
  adductor muscles of, 29, *29*, 86, *86*
    exercise for stretching, 87, *87*
    test for limited motion of, 29, *29*
  extensor muscles of, 84, *84*
    exercise precautions for, 50
    exercises for, 85, *85*
  flexor muscles of, 60, *60*
    exercises for stretching, 61, *61*
    test for limited motion of, 27, *27*
  lateral rotator muscles of, 30, *30*, 82, *82*, 86, *86*
    exercises for, 83, *83*
    exercises for stretching, 87, *87*
  medial rotator muscles of, 86, *86*
    exercises for stretching, 87, *87*
Hip joints, ligaments important to postural mechanics of, 47
Hollow chest, 19
Hooklying position, 44, *44*
Hook sitting position, 45, *45*

Iliacus, 60, *60*
Iliocostalis, 25, *25*, 56, *56*
Iliocostalis dorsi, 56, *56*
Iliocostalis lumborum, 56, *56*
Iliotibial band, 28, *28*
Indian sitting position, 45, *45*
Infraspinatus, 67, *67*
Inheritance, and posture, 1
Inspiration, primary muscles of, 75
Intercostals, 75, *75*
Interossei, dorsal, 92, *92*
Invertor muscle of foot, 90, *90*
  exercise for, 91, *91*

Joint(s), interphalangeal, extensor muscles of,
    exercises for stretching, 95, *95*
  knee, in body balance, 5
  metatarsal, adduction of, 21
  metatarsophalangeal, flexors of, 94, *94*
    exercises for, 95, *95*

Knee(s), extensor muscles of, 84, *84*
    exercises for, 85, *85*
  flexor muscles of, 31, *31*, 88, *88*
  hyperextended, 14, *14*
Knee joint, in body balance, 5
Kypholordosis, 13
Kyphosis, 13

Latissimus dorsi, 26, *26*, 70, *70*
Leg(s), bow, 20, *20*
  in evaluation of standing alignment, 14, *14*, 20, *20*
  knock knees, 20, *20*
  length of, measuring of, 36, *36*
  raising of, gravity and, *40*
Leg alignment. See *Alignment, of lower extremity,* and
    exercises for.

Lifting, correct and incorrect positions for, 104, *104*
  mechanics of, 101, *101*
Ligament(s), sacroiliac, 47, *47*
  sacrospinous, 47, *47*
  sacrotuberous, 47, *47*
Limited motion, evaluation of, 24–32, *24–32*
Locomotion, studies on, 79
Longissimus dorsi, 56, *56*
Long sitting position, 45, *45*
Longus capitis, 62, *62*
Longus colli, 62, *62*
Lordosis, 13
Lower extremity. See *Leg(s).*
Lumbar extensor muscles, 25, *25*, 56, *56*
  exercises for stretching of, 57–59, *57–59*
Lumbar spine, alignment of pelvic segment and, exercises for, 51–61, *51–61*
Lumbricales, 94, *94*
  exercises for, 95, *95*

Malalignment, 36
Mechanical balance, gravity line and, 4, *4*
Mesomorph, 8
Mobilization procedures, types of, 39–40
Motion, limited, evaluation of, 24–32, *24–32*
Muscle, weakness, 36
Muscles. See specific muscles and muscle groups; e.g.,
    Abductor digiti quinti and *Abductor muscles, of
    hip.*
  action potentials in, 5–6
  two-joint, passive tension in, 42
Muscle length, analysis of, in exercise program, 42
Muscle weakness, 36

Neck, extensor muscles of, 63, *63*
    exercises for axial extension of, 64–65, *64, 65*
  flexor muscles of, 62, *62*
    exercises for 64, *64*, 65, *65*

Obliquus externus abdominis, 50, *50*
Obliquus internus abdominis, 50, *50*
Obturator externus, 30, *30*, 82, *82*
Obturator internus, 30, *30*, 82, *82*
Oscillation, types of, 6

Pain, and exercise program, 38
Passive mobilization, procedures for, 39
Passive tension, in two-joint muscles, 42
Pectineus, 29, *29*, 86, *86*
Pectoralis major, 71, *71*
Pectoralis minor, 71, *71*
Pelvic area, anteroposterior rotary stresses on, 47
Pelvic segment, and lumbar spine, alignment of and exercises for, 51–61, *51–61*
Pelvis, determination of level of, 19, *19*
  examination of alignment of, planes of reference for, 46, *46*
  in evaluation of standing alignment, 19, *19*
  in body alignment, 46–48
Peroneus brevis, 96, *96*, 98
Peroneus longus, 96, *96*, 98
Pes planus, and foot pronation, 18
Physiological curves of spine, 3
Piriformis, 30, *30*, 82, *82*, 86, *86*
Planovalgus, 79
Postural scoliosis, 17, *17*
Posture, factors influencing, 1